Abnormal Speech

Originally published in 1939, it was only recently that serious study and attention had been given to disorders of speech and there was a growing demand for books dealing with the subject. *Abnormal Speech* deals concisely with the aetiology of the varied abnormalities of speech and discusses the treatment practised by experienced therapists at the time, successful in affecting permanent cures. It was now recognised that the causes and classification of speech disorders were fairly numerous, and that the essence of treatment consisted of discovering the nature and cause to apply the appropriate method of treatment. It was revised in 1950 in some part to account for the effects of the second world war on speech disorders. Today it can be read in its historical context.

This book is a re-issue originally published in 1939. The language used and views portrayed are a reflection of its era and no offence is meant by the Publishers to any reader by this re-publication.

I0127943

Abnormal Speech

E. J. Boome, H. M. S. Baines
and D. G. Harries

Routledge
Taylor & Francis Group
LONDON AND NEW YORK

First published in 1939
by Methuen & Co. Ltd
Second edition, revised 1950

This edition first published in 2025 by Routledge
4 Park Square, Milton Park, Abingdon, Oxon, OX14 4RN

and by Routledge
605 Third Avenue, New York, NY 10017

Routledge is an imprint of the Taylor & Francis Group, an informa business

© 1939, 1950 E. J. Boome, H. M. S. Baines and D. G. Harries

Publisher's Note
The publisher has gone to great lengths to ensure the quality of this reprint but points
out that some imperfections in the original copies may be apparent.

Disclaimer
The publisher has made every effort to trace copyright holders and welcomes
correspondence from those they have been unable to contact.

A Library of Congress record exists under LCCN: 40010204

ISBN: 978-1-032-93373-3 (hbk)
ISBN: 978-1-003-56583-3 (ebk)
ISBN: 978-1-032-93427-3 (pbk)

Book DOI 10.4324/9781003565833

ABNORMAL SPEECH

by

E. J. BOOME
T.D., M.B., CH.B., M.R.C.P., D.P.H., F.R.San.I., F.C.S.T.

FORMERLY PRINCIPAL ASSISTANT MEDICAL OFFICER, LONDON
COUNTY COUNCIL; CONSULTANT IN SPEECH THERAPY, LONDON
COUNTY COUNCIL

H. M. S. BAINES
F.C.S.T.

SPEECH THERAPIST, ROYAL SURREY COUNTY HOSPITAL, GUILDFORD; LECTURER IN
SPEECH THERAPY, ROYAL COLLEGE OF NURSING, AND BATTERSEA POLYTECHNIC;
FORMERLY SPEECH THERAPIST TO DAY CENTRES, WAR EMERGENCY AND MENTAL
HOSPITALS; HONORARY SPEECH THERAPIST, BELGRAVE HOSPITAL, LONDON

D. G. HARRIES
F.C.S.T.

SPEECH THERAPIST FOR DAY CENTRES AND MENTAL HOSPITALS;
LECTURER, LONDON COUNTY COUNCIL; FORMERLY HONORARY
SPEECH THERAPIST, BELGRAVE HOSPITAL, LONDON

SECOND EDITION REVISED AND RESET

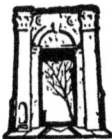

METHUEN & CO. LTD. LONDON
36 Essex Street, Strand, W.C.2

First Published March 1939
Second Edition, Revised, 1950

CATALOGUE NO. 3001/U

TO

THOSE WHO SUFFER

AND TO THOSE WHO TRY TO CURE

WE DEDICATE THIS BOOK

Preface

AS a member of the medical profession, and one who can no longer claim to be a young or even middle-aged man, I feel that I have had more than average opportunity of observing the suffering and trials to which humanity is so often submitted. It is my belief that most people pay dearly for their afflictions and too often lead lives of secret sorrow through no fault of their own. In the case of many of those troubled with abnormalities of speech this is certainly true; the whole personality, mental outlook and lives led by those so handicapped is deeply affected. Articulate speech is one of the most ancient and precious rights of man, language being one of the most potent forces in social life and civilization.

How often have intolerance and cruelty been the outcome of ignorance. Consider for a moment stammering, one of the most distressing and common forms of speech disorder and now recognized as being of nervous origin; how often has the nature of this condition been misunderstood. Little realizing the misery and torture the sufferer endures, relatives and others often subject him to constant fault-finding, discouragement, ridicule and other modes of ill-treatment so prejudicial to his happiness and prospects of improvement. Even when the stammerer is undergoing treatment from a speech therapist this critical attitude is often maintained. It is to be regretted that, speaking generally, members of the community have little psychological knowledge or understanding either of themselves or of their neighbours, and too frequently are incapable of censuring many of their own actions or appreciating the behaviour of others.

It is only within comparatively recent years that much serious study and attention has been given to disorders of speech, and there is a great and growing demand for books dealing with the subject. Hitherto, treatment has often been in the hands of quacks or those still clinging to obsolete methods which are based upon erroneous theories of the various causes of speech disturbances. The authors of this work, whilst realizing that further research may yet furnish added enlightenment upon the subject, deal concisely with the aetiology of the varied abnormalities of speech and discuss the modern treatment, as at present accepted, practised by experienced therapists successful in affecting permanent cures. It will be seen from a perusal of these pages that the causes and classification of speech disorders are now recognized as being fairly numerous. The essence of treatment consists in discovering the nature and cause of the particular faults and the utilization of appropriate methods.

The therapeutic value of relaxation for certain abnormalities of nervous origin is admitted. Relaxation, an almost forgotten art practised in bygone times (and one not so readily acquired as it might first be assumed), appears to be indicated in the treatment of all varieties of speech disorders, even where the speech defect under consideration is attributable to some organic condition.

There is an intimate relation between intelligence and the power of speech, so that it is not surprising to find abnormalities of speech prevalent among mental defectives. Social inefficiency is the recognized criterion of mental defectives certifiable under the Mental Deficiency Acts of 1913 and 1927, and speech therapy is being extensively practised in the institutions and colonies where the modern aim is to socialize (or render socially efficient), and to enable as many as possible to return to the community under suitable conditions ; this being, from an economic point of view, the only humane and practical policy of dealing with the gigantic social problem of mental deficiency. Social status and the possession of normal intelligence would appear to have little influence on the incidence of stammering.

The mechanism concerned in speech is complicated and the skilled speech therapist must be possessed of some acquaintance with physiology, anatomy, psychology and the value of suggestion. Moreover, since deafness, impaired vision, malformations, adenoids and other anomalies may all play some part in the causation and clinical picture presented by the patient, it follows that a physical examination becomes essential in all cases ; in addition, familiarity with the environment in which he lives is often of the utmost importance if the treatment is to be successful. It is vital that the treatment of stammering and other severe forms of speech disorder should always be in the hands of experts. Excellent work is now being done for the milder cases commonly found in schools and institutions by teachers and others who can also assist in carrying out the treatment even in some of the more severe cases.

The importance of the subject under consideration cannot be overestimated, and it is to be hoped that the authors' effort will be of some assistance to speech therapists and medical practitioners. It is also to be hoped that many others, including parents, will help in preventing, alleviating or eradicating some of the distressing conditions commonly to be observed among their fellow-creatures.

E. S. LITTELJOHN

The Manor
Epsom

Authors' Foreword

THERE has been so much controversy and difference of opinion on this subject in the past that we have now attempted to clarify the findings of others and to give the results of our own experience.

In view of the great interest that is taken in this subject throughout the country at the present time, we feel strongly that all results should be pooled with the hope that further progress will be made. It is to be hoped that all the therapists in this country will unite in this endeavour, and, in view of the unfortunate occurrences in other countries, we feel that the centre of speech therapy is now here.

We hope that this book will be of some help and guidance to Medical Superintendents of Certified Institutions and their staff, School Medical Officers, Speech Therapists, Teachers and Parents of children who are afflicted with speech troubles.

Abnormal speech may affect or be affected by the personality; and we have attempted to show this by examples and in the light of our experience. We would stress the fact that speech and behaviour are frequently in close relation, and in support of this thesis we have obtained valuable data from the very interesting work on this subject described by Dr. M. M. Lewis in his book *Infant Speech*.

In the course of this book we chiefly discuss the treatment of children, as one cannot forget that the child is father of the man, but if an adult has been unable to receive treatment when a child, we would like to point out that at no age is improvement impossible. The importance of early treatment cannot be too strongly emphasized; we see a number of cases who, had they had early treatment, would have been spared organic inferiority with its consequent mental anguish and suffering. Eminent ear, nose and throat authorities rightly emphasize the importance of early treatment in cleft palate cases.

We have long felt that the speech of the mentally defective has not been considered to be of sufficient importance, but it has now been realized that in placing these cases under guardianship or on licence the importance of intelligible speech cannot be ignored. The proof of this has been recognized by the appointment of speech therapists in the Certified Institutions for the Mentally Deficient with this end in view. We are indebted to Dr. E. S. Litteljohn, Medical Superintendent of the Manor, Epsom, for bringing out this point in his Preface.

We have received much guidance from the work of Miss Elsie Fogerty, the doyen of Speech Therapy, without whose inspiration this book would never have been written. We are also grateful to Dr. J. K. C. Laing, Medical Superintendent of Darenth Park Training Colony for the Mentally Deficient, and to Dr. Franklin Bicknell, for their constructive criticism and valuable advice.

E. J. B.
H. M. S. B.
D. G. H.

Foreword to the Second Edition

IN the spring of 1939 the first edition of this book was published. There is no need to remind our readers of the events which have taken place since that date. What effect has the war had on speech? We have been asked this question many times and it is most difficult to answer. Air raids, evacuation and family separations affected children in different ways. Some children undoubtedly developed a stammer as a result of their war experiences while others who suffered more severely were apparently unaffected. We are of the opinion that the nervous child was more adversely affected by evacuation, separation and shelter life (with its resulting lack of sleep) than by the actual air raids, but we did notice that a number of small children who were just beginning to speak, failed to develop the speech faculty after a shock. In some cases this was merely a retardation, and after a time the speech came normally; in others, however, the child developed a stammer or dyslalia.

Those of us who worked in War Emergency Hospitals where Service and Civilian cases were treated, found a large number of stammerers; these could be divided into different categories:

(*a*) Those who had always stammered.

(*b*) Those who had stammered as children and had ceased to do so but whose war experiences had caused a return of the stammer.

(*c*) Those who had a neuropathic inheritance, not necessarily that of stammering but any kind of neurosis (we think that stammering is not hereditary).

(*d*) Those who had never stammered before but owing to wounds or shock developed one.

We noticed in this category that the speech usually became normal after comparatively short treatment.

Much has been and is still being done to help those unfortunate patients suffering from head injuries, and in many cases speech has been restored completely or partially. If speech therapy has in any way helped these patients, surely that is a proof that a long-needed profession has justified its existence.

Speech therapists can play a great part in the treatment of aphasia, not only in helping the return of the actual speech but in aiding the whole well-being and happiness of the patient. We have had cerebral cases of patients of under 40 caused by overwork and overstrain associated with war conditions. The mental anxiety in these cases, especially where the patient is the bread-winner, induces further strain; it has been found that this anxiety can be alleviated by suggestion and muscular relaxation with corresponding benefit to condition caused by the lesion. It is a source of gratification to those of us who deal with these cases to see the general improvement in the mental attitude and confidence in the future.

We should like to thank the many friends, known and unknown, who have helped us by their appreciation and suggestions which we have endeavoured to carry out in this edition.

E. J. B.
H. M. S. B.
May 1949   D. G. H.

Contents

CHAPTER I

The Development of Normal Speech

The higher grade of development of ideas, of intellect and of reason which raise man above the brute, is intimately connected with the rise of language.

HAECKEL

SPEECH is not an exclusive prerogative of man. We have to recognize a long chain of evolution which stretches unbroken from the lowest to the highest stages. The higher gregarious animals need some means of communication; this is effected by touch, signs or sounds having a definite meaning. The song of the bird, the bark of the dog and the chirp of the cricket; all these are forms of animal speech. In addition the gibbon, an anthropoid ape, is said to be able to sing an octave. In his book, *A Naturalist on Lake Victoria*, Dr. Carpenter tells how he kept under observation two pet monkeys (Cercopithecus) and paid great attention to their 'speech'. He learnt to recognize thirteen distinct and different sounds and to attach a definite meaning to each; most of them were expressions of emotion, but not all; one indicated recognition; another was a cry for help, and a third, the most distinct, a hunting call.

Macneile Dixon says,

Animals are very much like ourselves in a hundred ways. We all know that, and there are many men who feel that the

2   I

affectionate relations between a dog and his master go further to establish the unity of living creatures than all the scientific doctrines. Of course men are animals, but how much more! Leave aside for a moment man's ethical and spiritual instincts, his ideals and aspirations. Consider only his obvious characteristics. The first witness to his astonishing ascendancy is the erect posture, his lifted gaze, contrasted with the hanging head of the quadruped. The second that he alone invented speech, the magic-working instrument, beside which all other inventions are childish toys. 'The *differentia* of man,' wrote the eminent anthropologist, Dr. Marett, 'the quality that marks him off from other animals, is undoubtedly his power of articulate speech. If language is ultimately the creation of intellect, yet hardly less fundamentally is the intellect a creation of language.' How ages meet! Homer knew it long ago. He spoke of μέροπες ἄνθρωποι beings endowed with, or dividing the voice, articulate speaking men.[1]

Speech, as we know it to-day, originally occurred some time during the age of the pithecanthropus (the Ape Man of Java) or the sinanthropus (the Pekin Man) and it is still in the process of evolution. The Australian aborigines are one of the oldest races extant.

There are many languages in Australia [writes Sollas] differing widely from one another both in structure and vocabulary. All are primitive, eminently plastic, with the promise of healthy growth for which the opportunity has now passed away. . . . As we might expect, their vocabulary is remarkably deficient in abstract and general terms; thus though every useful tree has its name, there is no word for tree in general; so with fish, there is a name for each kind that is good to eat, but for fish in general, only a phrase, such as 'food-in-water'. . . . Many of the Australian tribes could talk not only by speech, but by gesture. By an elaborate system of conventional signs they could carry on a simple conversation at a distance; a great convenience when there was any doubt whether an approaching party was of hostile or friendly intention.[2, 3]

---

[1] *The Human Situation.*   [2] Ancient Hunters.
[3] Hocart writes in the *Progress of Man*: 'Speech is far older than the common ancestor of all modern races. The conclusion can only

This 'system of conventional signs' is of inestimable value in helping the development of speech in children. It is necessary for our purpose to understand something of the process of this development. Speech is not merely the ability to utter articulate sound, but is the power of using words to express thoughts.

> The words of a man's mouth are as deep waters;
> The wellspring of wisdom is as a flowing brook.

Speech is a faculty that should develop normally as the child develops; any untoward happening that affects the personality during the more impressionable years may affect, either directly or indirectly, the behaviour

be that existing languages belong to a common stock. Otherwise we must suppose that the various branches of mankind gave up the language of their common ancestor and each created an entirely new one. Such breaks in evolution do not occur. Men never create new languages; they merely adapt old ones to new needs. Such artificial languages as Esperanto are exceptions that prove the rule: for they are based on existing languages, and the more they depart from them the more they fail. How is it that the comparative philologists have never been able to find any affinity between two neighbouring families like Aryan and Semitic, let alone Aryan and Iroquois? Because they have looked exclusively to words for evidence, they will not admit affinity unless they can identify with certainty a sufficient number of words. They will not admit that if the structure is nearly the same in two languages those languages must be closely related. The ways of expressing an idea, they argue, are limited, and so accidental resemblances must occur. But are not those ways limited precisely because all modern languages have so recently diverged from a common original? Distant species like dogs, monkeys, birds, ants, have some sort of speech, but their methods of expression are so remote from ours that we have no clue to their system; yet it is evident they can convey information, some of them detailed information.' Was this idea of a common stock held by the compilers of the Book of Genesis? 'And the whole earth was of one language and of one speech.'

and speech of the child. We cannot divorce speech and behaviour, but must consider, at every stage, the relation between the general behaviour of the child and his attitude as a speaker and listener.

Before we can use words to express our thought we must first have:

(*a*) The power to hear sounds.

(*b*) A conscious recognition of the object (or idea) for which the sound is a symbol.

(*c*) The ability to reproduce the sound, as the expression of the same object or idea.

The nervous mechanism concerned with speech consists of two pathways.

1. An afferent pathway with its prolongation to a higher conscious station, a connection between this conscious station and the motor speech centre, and thence—

2. An efferent pathway to the muscles concerned in phonation and articulation.

In addition to this we have every reason to believe that a more direct and subconscious connexion exists between the sensory and motor centres. Tredgold suggests that the nervous mechanism concerned in speech may be represented by the capital letter 'A', in which the side limbs denote the afferent and efferent paths respectively to and from consciousness, and the crosspiece the shorter subconscious connexion between the sensory and motor stations.

Thus disturbances of the speech faculty can take place in the sensory, intellectual or motor pathways. The great variation in the extent and nature of these defects is due to the fact that the impeding injury or disturbance may act upon:

(*a*) Parts of the brain concerned with the genesis of thought or the will to speak—the sensory pathways.

(*b*) Some parts of the nervous channels or the centres concerned with the actuation of speech—the intellectual or association pathways.

(*c*) The peripheral nerves and the organs concerned with articulation and vocalization—the motor pathways.

It will be seen that disturbances of the faculty of speech may, in some cases, be associated with the most marked alterations in the development of the intelligence, while in the others they may be represented by mere defective articulation or vocalization.

Stern's conclusions are that the child approaches speech along three paths:

1. The active expression of childish babble.
2. Unintelligent imitations.
3. Understanding what is said to him.

When these three actions, originally quite independent of each other, work together, real speech has begun. Sir Richard Paget says that speech is in fact the replacement of the muscular movements of expressive gestures by the specialized action of the laryngeal muscles.

Man has an inborn instinct for some form of articulate expression (as is seen in Stern's first stage of childish babble), but he does not speak by instinct. Articulate speech has to be learnt. This process of learning is mostly by imitation.

Speech arises as a form of expression. The child's first sounds denote comfort and discomfort; soon he is able to focus these expressions on pleasure or pain, for example, he will cry when he is hungry and make soft gurgling noises when his food arrives. Later he will make these sounds for their own sake and not as a form of expression; he will lie in his cot cooing and babbling, thus laying the foundation, by muscular memories, of aesthetic speech. If this state is interrupted by fear or repression, the speech may be delayed. It is from this moment that speech disorders may arise.

A child of 5 was brought to a clinic suffering from delayed speech. This condition his mother attributed to the fact that she had constantly stopped his cooing and babbling when a baby, owing to fear of her neighbours; she was at the time living in a one-room flat. In addition to this repression of the child's earliest sounds, it is highly probable that the mother refrained from the usual practice of playing with the child and helping him to build the foundations of vocabulary.

This natural instinct of parents to join in a child's babbling plays an important part in the acquirement of his mother tongue. The intervention by the adult into the child's babbling is valuable as the child imitates both phonetically and through intonation. Sometimes there appears to be considerable delay between the stimulus and the response, resulting in the child producing the word some time after he has heard it, in circumstances where it appears meaningless.[1] This is a normal stage in the growth of speech.

Thus the normal child goes through the following phases in developing the speech faculty:

1. He gives expression to the state of comfort and discomfort.

2. He responds to the expression of others.

3. He babbles.

4. He imitates and echoes.

5. He makes his first attempt at conversation (before any articulate words have been acquired) through the mother associating herself with the child's efforts by

[1] We would refer our readers to *Infant Speech* by M. M. Lewis, in which they will find this subject fully discussed.

alternating a recognized sound with the incoherent babble; for example, the baby's 'mm' followed by the mother's 'a' or 'i' becomes 'mamma' or 'mummy'.

6. He produces a word a long time after having heard it.[1]

These perfectly natural processes in preparation for speaking should be regarded in the same way as those for walking; namely, kicking, stretching, crawling, wobbling and stumbling; every stage has its meaning and helps towards development and co-ordination. It is when one stage is prolonged far beyond its normal course, due to some form of retardation, that it is considered to be a defect. In the normal child these stages are passed through and completed within the third year, his speech becomes more or less conventional and he has a vocabulary of several hundred words, with, probably, an occasional substitution of a difficult consonant by an easier one. The child uses a wrong word, notices its difference from that of other people, and is quick to imitate the correct sounds. In order to produce normal speech sounds the child must be able to hear them, feel the movements of his speech organs and, also, hear the sound he himself makes. If the child is deaf, careless or negligent, he fails to produce the sounds properly and does not even notice his mistakes.

During his early years the child passes through the stages of cooing and babbling, lalling, echolalia, metalalia or delayed imitation, and lisping; all these appear in the natural course of development. Most children pass through them happily and easily, but sometimes

---

[1] A consultant says that he spent some time in France as an infant; he returned to England before he was able to speak. When he did speak, certain French words appeared in his vocabulary.

through illness or shock one of the stages is prolonged unduly and the child may find it difficult to pass to the next stage, in the natural way, unless he is given some unobtrusive help.

If a child has difficulty in speech and through faulty associations produces a faulty sound, it is more than probable that the visual association will be incorrect.[1] In acquiring the faculty of speech a child must hear and understand before he is able to produce a coherent sound.

NORMAL SPEECH DEMANDS:

(a) A Mental content to be expressed.
(b) An acquired vocabulary and language.
(c) Utterance.

As the child develops he acquires the use and co-ordination of these three, and through listening, imitation by association and expression the speech faculty is developed.

The province of Speech Therapy is the study and rehabilitation of those cases in which, through congenital or acquired defect, the child is incapable of carrying out this process up to the level of his general speech environment. We call the obstacles to this normal development, Speech Defects.

Any difficulty in the development of speech, however slight, is almost bound to affect the personality of the child. Speech is the external expression of self, and a child will differentiate between what he considers his outward behaviour and his true self; he will accept correction in the first case cheerfully enough, but will resent deeply any interference with his individuality.

The object of the therapist should be to draw out and

[1] This subject is discussed in Chapter VII.

develop the latent power of the child and to inspire him with a desire to reach the goal where his language adequately expresses every thought that he wishes to utter. The aim of this book is to show that it is possible to adjust the personality of the patient to a positive attitude to his difficulties, and to help him to acquire the desire to cure himself.

CHAPTER II

Disorders of Speech : Dyslalia and Dysarthria

..., but what is it that hath burnt thine heart?
For thy speech flickers like a blown-out flame.

SWINBURNE

IN a former edition we attempted to divide disorders of speech into three categories, functional, organic and psychogenic, but at the same time explaining that these divisions were not comprehensive and that many defects of speech came under two or even three headings; so a lisp might be functional, organic, psychogenic or all three.

Present-day authorities are inclined to use the following terms:

Dyslalia. All types of articulatory defects due to functional weakness.

Dysarthria. Defects due to injury, malformation, disease or degeneration of the organs of speech.

DYSLALIA

A defect of articulate speech (Stein)

I. GENERAL DYSLALIA

Also known as Delayed Speech

This term is used when the speech faculty does not appear at the normal stage. It may be due to many causes, the most serious of which are mental deficiency and congenital deafness. The lack of speech, however, may be due to general debility following a severe illness, operation, accident, shock or to pure laziness. Therefore it can be seen that delayed speech may result from physical, mental, or psychological causes.

Children suffering from delayed speech are sometimes mentally unstable; because they lack the power to express their emotion in words, they try to get the attention they want by appearing restless, impatient, bad-tempered and destructive. They seem to be unable to concentrate, and one is sometimes puzzled to know whether this is a sign of true instability or a defence reaction. Often what seems to the parent and teacher mere naughtiness is in reality an inhibition caused through failure to express their thought normally in speech. As the speech progresses these distressing symptoms gradually disappear.

Sometimes these children are very sensitive and cry easily; in most cases they are very affectionate, and if the teacher can gain their confidence by giving them definite small responsibilities, a great deal of their shyness is dispelled. In every case it is advisable for the child to go to school, as the contact with other children helps him towards self-adjustment.

Cases have come to our notice recently of young children who have temporarily lost their speech after a severe air raid; these children had either just begun to speak (1-2 years), or else were speaking quite fluently (3-4 years), but the shock temporarily took away their power of speech, as the habit was not completely established. In some cases a stammer ensued, and in others a severe dyslalia: in the very young children the speech was delayed, but eventually became quite normal.

2. SIMPLE DYSLALIA

Formerly known as Lisping

The lisper has usually a constitutional dislike of accuracy in any movement; he has difficulty in performing the simplest hand exercises with precision. A lisper is often deficient in physical energy and thinks slowly in consequence. He has a feeling of inadequacy and is either afraid or has no desire to strike out for himself; he seems content to exist but not to live. If his ambition can be aroused and his health improved (the terms are probably synonymous) the speech will improve rapidly, and, if the child is merely dull or backward but not deficient, his mental powers will show equal progress.

(*a*) SIGMATISM. *S*. The commonest form of lisping is difficulty with the 's' sound (sigmatism). In 's' the tip of the tongue must be placed behind the top or bottom teeth, the sides of the tongue are raised forming a narrow channel through which the air passes. The chief faults are as follows:

1. Spurious 'TH'. The tip of the tongue is between the teeth damming the channel and diverting the air to form a hissed 'th' (see formation of 'th' below).
2. Lateral 'S'. The channel is flattened causing the air to escape at the sides of the tongue. The sound produced is akin to the unvoiced Welsh 'Ll'.
3. Uvula 'S'. A guttural fricative. The sound is produced in the throat, the tongue flattened and the resultant sound resembles the German 'ich'.
4. Thickened 'S'. The channel is flattened, the sides of the tongue are pressed against the upper

molars. The sound is similar to that of 'sh' but the omission of lip movement gives it a dull lifeless tone.

5. Nasal 'S'. A voiceless 'n'. Without the necessary tongue movements the air is directed through the nose. In cases of cleft palate this sound sometimes resembles an exaggerated 'h'.

6. Palatal Stop. Owing to the faulty approximation of the tongue muscles, too much effort is made and the sound changed from a continuant to a stop, i.e. 't' is produced instead of 's'.

(b) FAULTY. *TH.* Another common error in lisping is that of the faulty 'th'. 'f' and 'v' are substituted for voiced and unvoiced 'th'. In the sound 'th' the tip of the tongue is placed between the teeth and drawn smartly backwards. Owing to inertness or to mistakes in hearing it is found easier to approximate the upper teeth to the lower lip and the fricative 'f' or 'v' ensues.

3. MULTIPLE DYSLALIA
Often known as Lalling

There are three stages in the development of the speech faculty, the sounds which the child makes for his own amusement, his attempt to use these sounds in imitation of the words he hears, and finally his successful reproduction of these sounds into words. The child at first makes no attempt at the more difficult sounds, then attempts them unsuccessfully and finally he reaches the stage of mastering them. In the second stage, which may be of short or long duration, the child's mental capacity is in advance of his muscular memory. In any difficulty he either substitutes a completely different sound, attempts a sound like it, or leaves it out altogether. A child of 2 called gloves 'belaws'. This may be due to:

(a) The breath-stop 'g' is substituted for an easier breath-stop 'b'.

(b) A vowel is placed before the 'l' as an occlusive followed by 'l' causes difficulty in many cases.

(c) The 'v' is elided and the vowel AW (ɔ:), found easier than the subordinate (ʌ).

In the normal child this is a passing phase, as he quickly realizes that he is not speaking like other people and adapts himself to the standard pronunciation. It is when this substitution is carried on beyond its normal stage that it comes under the category of defective speech; often it is the faculty of listening that is faulty, the child has not learnt to focus his attention to recognize and produce the correct sound.

According to many modern writers on psychology, it is the mother who is responsible for all faults which develop in her children. Without concurring wholly with this pessimistic view of the mental capacity of British motherhood, it is unfortunately true to say that this form of speech is often found in the over-fussed and over-indulged child.

All movement is generated by energy. The amount of energy needed can be calculated by a well-balanced brain; over- or under-estimation of the required energy will result from either a tense or sluggish brain and produce an unrhythmic movement. The laller, like his near relation the lisper, fails to estimate the energy required and this faulty estimation is probably the cause of his omission of the final consonants and almost universal difficulty with the 'r' sound.

(*a*) SUBSTITUTION OF CONSONANTS. In cases of lalling, the following substitutions are common:

1. The interchanging of the front and back lingual breath stops 't', 'd', for 'k' and 'g', e.g. 'tind dirl' for 'kind girl'.
2. 'y' for 'l', e.g. 'yady' for 'lady'.
3. 'l' for 'y', e.g. 'lellow' for 'yellow'.

The 'l' sound is produced by the tip of the tongue touching the hard palate immediately behind the top teeth and allowing the breath to pass between them and the sides of the tongue. The 'y' sound is produced by the tip of the tongue touching the lower teeth-ridge, the back raised and the sides pressing against the top teeth. The breath passes through this diminished space, and the definite pressure against the top teeth almost causes a breath stop.

In the substitution 'y' for 'l' the tip of the tongue fails to approximate correctly against the hard palate and to compensate for this the rest of the tongue makes a clumsy movement against the top teeth.

In the opposite fault 'l' for 'y' the sides of the tongue are inert and the tip only is used. This fault usually occurs when a true 'l' follows.

(*b*) OMISSION OF FINAL CONSONANTS. In addition to these faults, there is a tendency to omit the final sound of any word which ends with two consonants, the effort required for their production being too great for the child's limited capacity.

The laller might be described as the champion assimilator and simplifier of consonants. In standard English speech it is not only permissible but correct to simplify consonant groups, but there are certain rules governing this simplification, for example, although we may drop the 't' in 'Christmas', in 'last man' the final 't' should be spoken. The laller follows his own sweet will in these matters with the result that his speech is often unintelligible.

4. RHOTACISM

One theory maintains that in the early stages of all languages the 'r's' were tongue trilled, this required effort which was gradually lessened in most languages. In England it became untrilled or was completely dropped, in other countries it became an uvula or throat 'r'. In France and Germany the tongue 'r' remained in the country, the throat 'r' is found in the towns.

In Southern English 'r' the tongue is raised, the tip is curled back resting on the hard palate; the air passing between this narrow passage causes the friction necessary for the production of this sound. The position of the tongue is the same for the trilled and untrilled sound but in the former the vibrations are more numerous. In Southern English the 'r' is only pronounced before a vowel, e.g. in 'pray' but not in 'pearl'. If a word ends in 'r' followed by a vowel, the 'r' is usually sounded, e.g. 'more and more'.

In addition to the standard Southern English 'r' the following variations are often heard in different parts of the country:

1. Trilled 'r'. Native to Scotland, Northern England and Ireland.
2. Uvula 'r'. This is not a sound found in standard English, but is frequently heard in Durham and Northumberland, and is known as the Northumbrian burr. Professor W. Ripman says, 'It

is a sound admirably produced by most babies, especially when lying on the lap and with their heads hanging back. The tongue "r" on the other hand gives them much trouble, and consequently appears rather late in their speech.' [1]

3. West Country 'r' is untrilled. The tip of the tongue is curled very far back producing the sound heard in Devonshire. The fact that this sound is also heard in America suggests a theory that it is an inheritance from the Pilgrim Fathers, so many of whom were natives of the West.

THE ERROR OF 'R'

1. 'w' for 'r'. Owing to the weakness of tongue-tip muscles the lips compensate and produce an effect like 'w', e.g. wabbit for rabbit.
2. 'l' for 'r'. The blade of the tongue is pressed against the hard palate, e.g. led for red.
3. 'y' for 'r'. The tongue tip is inert. The sides of the tongue being used instead, e.g. yound for round.

CLUTTERING

Hurried, jumbled speech. This defect is usually found in young children; the small child has more ideas than he has capacity for utterance; the error may also appear at puberty. Judging by the numerous German writers on the subject of cluttering Kerr has arrived at the conclusion that this defect is of more common occurrence in Germany than in England. Cluttering must not be confused with stammering, although with wrong treatment

[1] *The Sounds of Spoken English.*

the clutterer may easily become a stammerer. The clutterer speaks better the more he thinks about his speech, the stammerer, the less he thinks about it. Cluttering is a symptom of nervous haste, stammering of nervous fear.

IDIOGLOSSIA

This defect is considered by some authorities to be a form of aphasia, by others to be a form of dyslalia.

In idioglossia the consonantal substitutions are so extensive that the child appears to have a language peculiar to himself. This condition is frequently found among the mentally defective. It is also occasionally found in very young children of normal intelligence, and is then probably due to delayed imitation.

As this is a retardation rather than a defect, any exercises that will help in the development of the speech faculty should be given. Sense training apparatus and pictures are most helpful to give the child a feeling of the right use of words. It is important to stimulate his interest in his surroundings in order to counteract the sense of isolation which his speech gives him. This isolation may be deliberate, induced by a desire to live in a world of his own.

Sometimes idioglossia occurs in the youngest child of a family, especially if one or more of the older children are of a dominating nature. It is noticeable that as a rule one of the older children, understanding the language, acts as interpreter for the younger and speaks for him (cf. Horace Hemsley).

A sense of independence must be instilled and the child encouraged to speak for himself.

ECHOLALIA

The meaningless repetition of words and phrases

This disturbance occurs in nervous disorders and low-grade mentally defectives. A very nervous child may have a mild form of this trouble, and the general health and behaviour should be carefully watched. It can also occur in a mild degree in anyone suffering from physical exhaustion and has been known in cases of cerebral tumour.

Tredgold says:

This condition is not very common and is somewhat difficult to explain. I am disposed to think that it may be due to the child's consciousness being so swamped or occupied (by emotions of fright or anxiety, in some cases at the presence of a stranger or unaccustomed surroundings) that auditory sounds only reach a subconscious motor centre, and are thence immediately translated into speech. There is, in fact, a short-circuiting of the nerve current. This condition, as far as I am aware, does not occur in persons of normal mental development, although it is, of course, by no means uncommon for a person to speak who is totally unconscious of his surroundings. Many normal children, whilst busily engaged in some occupation, will repeat words which are pronounced near them, without seemingly understanding the words or being aware of the fact that they have copied them. It is presumably by a similar subconscious mechanism that echolalia occurs.[1]

APHASIA

A disorder of speech resulting from lesions of special speech centres in the cerebral cortex, of association fibres deep to those centres, and also from lesions of the motor cortical centres and paths connecting them with the muscles of articulation.

Formerly the term aphasia was used to denote the inability to express thought by means of speech which

[1] *Mental Deficiency.*

follows certain diseases of the brain; in recent years it has obtained a wider significance and may now be defined as the loss of the faculty of interchanging thought, without any affection of the intellect or will.

Interchange of thought involves:

(a) The expression of mental processes by means of conventional symbols, i.e. gesture, speech and writing.

(b) The understanding of these symbols.

The interchange of thought may be interrupted by derangement of any one of these processes. In the former case, the change affects the mechanism conducting from the mental idea to the symbol, which is often termed the motor symbol process; in the latter there is an alteration in the mechanism conducting impulses from the symbol to the motor idea, often called the sensory process. There is therefore a motor and a sensory aphasia.

MOTOR APHASIA. A loss of the memory of the co-ordinated movements necessary for the formation of symbols. The patient although able to recognize an object is unable to name it, and, although understanding a question, is unable to reply. He may be able to show acquiescence or dissent by means of gesture, but in most cases this power is absent.

SENSORY APHASIA. A loss of memory of the meaning of symbols. The patient can speak without understanding his own words or detecting any error that he may make. In some cases he is unable to understand the spoken word; in many, he can write and read correctly.

It is not within the province of this book to discuss in detail those disturbances which are known as aphasic disorders. The work in this subject is still in the research stage, and what was considered fact a few years ago has, in some cases, been questioned, and in others contradicted. We include a short list of the better-known types of aphasia, but it is almost impossible to divide them faithfully under the headings Motor and Sensory, as in many cases both processes are affected.

(a) ALALIA. (i) Inability to articulate by paralysis of the muscles of speech or an affection of the larynx.

(ii) Hysterical Mutism. Loss of speech due to psychological causes. With no organic injury.

(b) ALEXIA. Word blindness. A form of Aphasia in which the patient is unable to recognize written or printed characters.

(i) *Motor Alexia.* Inability to read aloud what is written or printed, although it is comprehended.

(ii) *Musical Alexia.* Loss of the ability to read music.

(iii) *Optic Alexia.* Inability to comprehend written or printed words.

(c) AGRAPHIA. Inability to express ideas by writing.

(i) *Absolute Agraphia.* A variety in which no letters can be formed.

(ii) *Acoustic Agraphia.* Loss of capacity to write from dictation.

(iii) *Amnemonica Agraphia.* A form in which letters can be written, but without conveying any meaning.

(iv) *Atactica Agraphia.* That form in which letters cannot be formed from lack of muscular co-ordination.

(v) *Motor Agraphia.* Inability to recall the movements of the hand necessary in writing.

(vi) *Musical Agraphia.* Pathological loss of the ability to write musical notes.

(vii) *Optic Agraphia.* Inability to copy writing, but ability to write from dictation.

(viii) *Verbal Agraphia.* A variety in which a number of words without meaning can be written.

(d) AGNOSIA. An impairment of the Sensory pathways which results in an inability to recognize familiar objects. This disturbance may arise in any of the Sensory pathways and may be of short duration, for example: the sense of smell or taste sometimes becomes temporarily inactive as the result of illness.

(e) AMNESIA. (Forgetfulness.) Inability to recall particular words or groups of words.

(f) ANARTHRIA. Complete absence of normal articulate speech, whether whispered or spoken. This is due to trauma, inflammation, degeneration or to peripheral nerve lesions.

(g) APHEMIA. A form of motor Aphasia in which the patient is unable to articulate words and sentences due to an injury in the nerve centre.

CONGENITAL AUDITORY IMPERCEPTION

A disorder of speech in which the child makes an attempt, usually imperfect, to imitate what he hears spoken, but does not understand the meaning of the words. It is ascribed to developmental failure of the speech centres.

DISORDERS OF PHONATION

1. APHONIA

Complete loss of voice

This may arise from pathological conditions of the larynx. It is in some cases a symptom of hysteria or of anxiety neurosis; it may also result from a severe shock, and a second shock may restore speech.

2. DYSPHONIA

Impairment of voice

This may be functional, hysterical or pathological.

(a) FUNCTIONAL NASALIZATION (RHINOPHONIA). A nasal tone in speaking. In debilitated or men- tally defective children, the soft palate, though anatomically perfect, may fail to perform its function in speaking. This may be yet another case where the child is too lazy or too careless to make the necessary effort for co-ordinated speech.

(b) HUSKINESS. Harsh whispered tone caused by slack- ness or spasticity of the muscles of phonation. It may be due to a pathological condition of the larynx. It is often found in nervous children.

(c) THROATY TONE. This is caused by the constriction of the muscles of the front of the throat and the back of the tongue, due to too much attention being concentrated on the larynx instead of on the two ends of the vocal apparatus, i.e. breath- ing and the orbicular muscles.

(*d*) PHONASTHENIA. Weak whispered tone due to nervousness. In moments of stress, shy children (especially girls) exhibit symptoms of this trouble. In the mentally deficient it sometimes appears to be a permanent condition (cf. Huskiness).

(*e*) GLOTTAL SHOCK. The vocal cords are pressed together instead of being approximated and the breath comes out jerkily, producing a sound resembling a cough before a vowel.

In certain cases this sound is substituted for a consonant in the middle of the word, e.g. wa'er for water, bu'er for butter. Although found in many functional disorders, this defect is very common in palatal troubles. It may also appear in psychogenical disturbances.

In an excellent chapter in *Speech in Childhood*, Seth and Guthrie state that hoarseness is due in some cases to excessive crying in small children, and in others to singing beyond the capacity of the voice. They also say 'not only may children injure their voices in singing or in shouting when at play, but the habitual tone employed in conversational speech may be pitched too high or too low'

Many promising voices are spoiled through this tendency to over-sing their capacity. A very musical girl with a singing voice of exceptional clarity and beauty was allowed to sing at school concerts and to undertake many public engagements, until at the age of 18 her voice was beyond training. In addition to this strain her habit of over-loud every-day speech was probably a contributory factor to the breakdown of her singing voice. Children's voices have also been ruined through parents allowing them to speak in a whining pseudo-affectionate manner.

DYSARTHRIA

DEAFNESS

The most important congenital disorder affecting speech is deafness; before a child can speak correctly, he must not only hear what is said to him but be able to hear the sound he himself produces. There are several types of deafness, namely:

(a) CORTICAL DEAFNESS. Loss of hearing as a result of destruction of the auditory arrival platforms, but with no disease of the ears or auditory nerves.

(b) MIND DEAFNESS. (Auditory Agnosia.) Loss of the ability to understand the meaning of sounds of the environment, although they are heard.

(c) WORD DEAFNESS. (i) Acquired—Loss of the ability to understand the spoken word. (ii) Developmental (Congenital). Difficulty in learning to understand the spoken word.

(d) REGIONAL DEAFNESS. Lowered acuity of hearing in a part only of the normal range of pitch. This may include chiefly the lower range, when it is called *Bass* Deafness, but more commonly the higher range is affected, resulting in High Frequency Deafness, i.e. an inability to hear the following sounds: S, Z, F, TH, SH, CH. The child's hearing may be perfectly normal in every other way, but to these sounds he is deaf.[1]

(e) PERIPHERAL DEAFNESS. Deafness due to disease of

[1] *The Child's Hearing for Speech*, Mary D. Sheridan, M.D., L.R.A.M.

the ear or auditory nerve as contrasted with that due to brain lesions as described above.

PALATAL DEFECTS

For all sounds, except the nasal m, n and ng, the velum or soft palate is raised into position against the pharyngeal wall, thus closing the passage from nose and throat; if this is not done the speech has a dull nasal quality. In the case of the occlusives, or breath stops, p, b, t, d and k, g, the lips or the tongue close the frontal air passage, the air which accumulates under some pressure is released by the lips or through the mouth. If the velum is dropped before this release, the explosion occurs through the nose, resulting in a peculiar 'snorting' sound. This action of the velum, an organ over which we have no direct control, plays a very important part in speech.

The chief defects are:

(a) CLEFT PALATE SPEECH. This speech varies with extent of the injury, it may range from some difficulty with sibilants accompanied by a nasal voice to almost complete incoherence due to excessive nasality (rhinolalia aperta) and mispronunciation of vowels and consonants.

(b) MALFORMED PALATE. The speech closely resembles that of cleft palate and may be due to excessive height of the palatal arch or to shortness of the uvula.

(c) ATROPHY, PARALYSIS AND PARESIS OF THE VELUM.

(i) Atrophy is a wasting away of the muscles due to lack of use.

(ii) Paralysis the loss of movement and sensation.

(iii) Paresis the loss of movement only.

Paralysis and Paresis may result from diphtheria.

(d) SUB-MUCOUS CLEFT. A fissure in the bony structure which affects the voice in the same manner as cleft palate.

(e) POST-ADENOID SPEECH. (Rhinolalia clausa.) When adenoids are present the closure is made against them; after their removal the movement of the velum sometimes remains the same, leaving a gap between it and the rear wall of the parynx, whereby all sounds become nasal.

OBSTRUCTED NASAL PASSAGES

A condition found temporarily in severe colds. The turbinates become swollen and the nasal cavities are more or less closed; the obstruction deprives the sounds of their peculiar ring:

'm' sounds like 'b'.
'n'   ,,   ,, 'd'.

Permanently enlarged turbinates or a deflected septum may cause a similar result.

The speech of obstructed nasal passages is the opposite to that of cleft palate. The nasalization of cleft palate consists in adding nasal tones to sounds where they do not occur; the denasalization from obstruction consists in eliminating nasal tones when they should be present.

TONGUE DEFECTS

If the tongue is too thick, too small, too clumsy, or is injured, there are likely to be resulting inaccuracies of speech.

(a) HEMIATROPHY OF THE TONGUE. The sides of the tongue may be unequal, the surface grooved and fibrillary twitchings present. This may or may not affect speech.

(*b*) TONGUE TIE. This condition is extremely rare, although in the past it was considered common and the membrane was unnecessarily incised. A distinguished surgeon at a London Children's Hospital states that he has only seen one case requiring surgical treatment. There is still an antiquated belief that tongue tie causes stammering.

JAW DEFECTS

The chief defects are overshot and underhung jaw.

(i) OVERSHOT JAW. The oral resonance is diminished and the vowels thereby affected; consequently it is difficult to adjust the tongue correctly for the sibilants.

(ii) UNDERHUNG JAW. The projection of the upper teeth causes the lower lip to impede the tongue in producing the sounds: t, d, th, s, sh, and their compounds.

DENTAL IRREGULARITIES

In some cases a cause of sigmatism; this difficulty with the 's' may begin during the period of second dentition. If care is not taken the trouble may continue and the fault which started as a mechanical difficulty may become a habit, ending in a functional defect.

Joan van Thal recently examined a number of children undergoing orthodontic treatment with the object of ascertaining whether the state of their teeth had in any way affected their speech. She says:

> In spite of the high proportion of grossly erroneous and mildly defective speech found amongst these cases of dental anomaly we are not justified in jumping to the conclusion that the state of dentition is solely responsible for the faulty speech. Control tests on the children with normal dental formation gave a very high percentage of stridency on sibilants, and some mild interdentalism

too. There is sufficient evidence available to prove that adaptability and skill in the use of the tongue compensate for many dental malformations. It is where tongue control is inadequate that we get such a great number of lispers. Where we have this faulty tongue control, either alone or coupled with auditive difficulties, faulty dentition is an added complication. It may influence, but it does not cause the defect of speech.

It should be noted that all the children examined by me were subjected to tests for tongue movement apart from speech as well as to the speech tests, and that 86 per cent were found to have unsatisfactory, if not actually in each case bad, tongue control. This investigation seems to confirm what has already been affirmed by Froeschels and the Vienna School, namely, that while bad dentition has an unfavourable influence on speech we are not justified in regarding it as the actual cause of such articulatory defects as lisping; the cause lies rather in the faulty innervation of the lingual muscles.

Finally, it must be borne in mind that in all disorders of speech there may be functional and psychological as well as organic causes. For therapeutic purposes even the simplest form of such a defect as lisping has its psychological aspects.[1]

We have attempted to describe briefly the commoner forms of functional and organic disorders of speech. In a later chapter we discuss those disorders which are disturbances of the nervous system and are of psychogenic origin.

[1] *The Relationship between Faults of Dentition and Defects of Speech* (reprinted from 'The Proceedings of the Second International Congress of Phonetic Sciences').

CHAPTER III

Treatment of Speech Disorders : Dyslalia and Dysarthria

Never let the child lose heart; for once he has lost heart he has lost everything.

CYRIL BURT

THE essential factor in good speech is co-ordination. It is of the first importance to remember the whole personality of the patient in the treatment of the particular symptom. In order to accomplish this all exercises given should be based on relaxation and rhythm.

It has been found of inestimable value to begin all treatment by muscular relaxation; this physical ease leads to mental control. In addition to the organic defect there is often a superimposed tension, which may show itself either in a strained anxious appearance or in a lethargic attitude. These apparently opposite faults have the same origin and may be relieved by relaxation.

All movements connected with speech must be:

1. Easy—no strain.
2. Smooth—no jerk.
3. Purposeful—under control of the will.

In order to obtain control, complete muscular relaxation is necessary.

The aim of all exercise is:

1. Flexibility
2. Rhythm   }Control.
3. Co-ordination

Rhythm is the fundamental law of movement, as gravitation is the fundamental law of stability. Every action must take place through a certain space, during a certain time, and with a certain degree of force. When space, time and force are properly measured, under the direction of a definite intention, the result is a rhythmic movement. When rhythm is used to make definite patterns of sound, colour, line or words, we get music, art, or poetry. People often mistake these patterns for rhythm itself, and confuse 'time' in music or 'metre' in poetry with rhythm. These things do not become rhythmical till they express meaning or intention.

Speech is movement, and is therefore subject to all conditions which produce good rhythmic movement, namely, clear and definite mental intention and exact muscular control. Hence the need for intelligent and scientific practice.

There is no such thing as 'natural' speech. All speech is acquired or taught movement, but careless or pedantic speech alike will be found to be lacking in the true qualities of rhythm.[1]

Speech is a highly co-ordinated process. It entails the synchronization of the organs of speech, and of hearing with understanding. Before a child speaks he must have laid the foundation for it by the muscular practice of cooing and babbling; he must also have dimly perceived the association of his sounds with people or objects. His speech must grow naturally as the outward and audible sign of his inward development. A child suffering from defective speech often finds concentrated attention difficult owing to lack of co-ordination; in many cases this failure to concentrate is due to fatigue caused by excessive misdirected energy. The child is conscious that

[1] *First Notes on Speech Training*, Elsie Fogerty.

he is not speaking like other people, and this self-consciousness causes either muscular tension or a lack of
concentration, both of which are a constant drain on
the child's energy. It is essential to stop this waste of
energy before any constructive speech work is begun.
As the child learns to relax his muscles and finds in
consequence that he is able to do many things with his
body of which he was previously incapable, he gains
confidence through his growing power of co-ordination,
and begins to realize that speech is a movement.
Through simple rhythmic exercises he acquires flexibility of the muscles under the direction of the will;
these co-ordinated movements can grow into significant
gestures and lead to simple dramatization of nursery
rhymes. The child's imagination is thus stimulated, he
has the desire for self-expression and is ready for speech.

DYSLALIA

I. GENERAL DYSLALIA—DELAYED SPEECH

In the treatment of this condition it is helpful to use
all the sense training exercises, such as pictures, puzzles
for shape, size and colour, elementary weaving and, in
fact, any apparatus used in the nursery school and
kindergarten adapted to the child's special need. A boy
of 5 learnt his first lesson of obedience with a pair of
reins. Walking, marching and skipping to music is both
helpful and amusing to the child.

Under no circumstances must the child attempt to
say a word of which he does not understand the meaning. After learning objects and their names, he can
learn qualities. In feeling that the ball is round he
learns the quality of roundness, in touching velvet and
sandpaper he realizes the opposite qualities of smooth-
ness and harshness. In all these exercises the child is

interested and amused, and thus the will to speak is stimulated.

Sometimes, in response to the necessary stimulus, the speech suddenly appears in a perfect form and the child, who has hitherto been dumb, is able to present his ideas in well-formed sentences. More often when the speech function is late in developing, it appears in the mutilated form of lalling and lisping.

2. SIMPLE DYSLALIA—LISPING

(*a*) SIGMATISM. As this fault is the result of a misdirected breath, it is helpful to begin treatment with blowing exercises. A very simple and efficacious method is for the child to place his little finger against his closed teeth and blow, the sound produced is 's'. When he has heard himself make this sound and felt the position of his tongue, let him open his teeth into the position of 'AH', repeating this exercise without moving the tip of the tongue from the teeth.

Sometimes it is helpful to use a drinking straw balanced between the teeth as a guide for the breath; the child may also find it amusing to practise blowing down a small hollow key.[1]

(*b*) FAULTY 'TH'. Although the commonest of defects, especially among London children, it is usually one of the easiest to correct. Place the finger in front of the lips, let the tip of the tongue touch the finger and be drawn smartly back across the top teeth; the sound is made as the tongue is drawn back.

3. MULTLE DYSLALIA—LALLING

Baby talk is a natural phase in the development of the speech function; but, what is a natural condition

---

[1] Cf. *Cleft Palate Speech*, J. van Thal; *Speech in Childhood*, Seth and Guthrie.

4

at 18 months becomes a marked defect at 6 years. The arrested development of the speech function is the cause of this defect; the elision, substitution and assimilation the result. First treat the laller, then the lalling.

SUBSTITUTION OF CONSONANTS ('t' and 'd' for 'k' and 'g', 'y' for 'l', etc.). The phonetic position of each sound should be shown, the child made to see his movements in a looking-glass and to feel the contact of the back, sides and tip of the tongue. If the child places his finger on his top lip and under his chin he is able to feel, and consequently visualize, the correct positions for the front and back breath stops.

OMISSION OF FINAL CONSONANTS. This usually occurs in words ending with a breath stop, in a combination of consonants or sometimes in a nasal consonant. Example: go' for got, pas' for past, I' going for I'm going, etc.

These faults are largely due to slowness in changing the breath direction. Exercises for breath direction, for flexibility of the tongue, lips and jaw should be given. The speech sounds should be practised singly and in pairs in conjunction with rhythmic hand movements.

4. RHOTACISM

In the previous chapter we mentioned that the failure to estimate the required energy is the cause of the almost universal difficulty with the 'r' sound experienced by the laller. The lack of skill, both motor and sensory, make it wellnigh impossible for the child to master the fine adjustments necessary for the vibrations required. The tongue must be in such perfect condition that the child can feel the co-ordinated movements.

Exercise to strengthen the muscles of the tongue should be given, the child should be encouraged to feel the sensations in the tongue during these exercises.

CLUTTERING

This defect is usually found in the young child with a quick brain whose ideas are in advance of his unskilled articulatory apparatus. The treatment should be, relaxation for the nervous haste, rhythmic movements for the excessive speed and co-ordinated speech exercises for the jumbled words.

IDIOGLOSSIA

As this is a retardation rather than a defect, any exercises that will help in the development of the speech faculty should be given. Sense training apparatus and pictures are most helpful to give the child a feeling of the right use of words. It is important to stimulate his interest in his surroundings in order to counteract the sense of isolation which his speech gives him. This isolation may be deliberate, induced by a desire to live in a world of his own. Sometimes idioglossia occurs in the younger of two children, especially if the elder is of a dominating nature; the older child understanding the language of the younger, speaks for him. A sense of independence must be instilled and the child made to speak for himself.

ECHOLALIA

In its extreme form this disorder is usually found among the low-grade mentally defective, but in a mild form it may be associated with extreme nervousness.

This condition will be alleviated if the nervous condition is improved.

APHASIA

We wish to emphasize the importance of the preliminary handling of the patient. In some cases the stressing of the speech side too soon may cause considerable mental irritation to the patient. He must not 'be taught to speak' until he is ready. It is much safer to give the patient a course of relaxation before attempting to do any speech work. When the mental anxiety and irritation is relieved by relaxation, the patient can then be given muscular exercises of the articulatory apparatus. The movement of unparalysed muscles may help to alleviate the paresis of those damaged.

If the patient can be taught the positions of the speech sounds through the sense of feeling he may recover the muscular memory of those sounds.

The nature and degree of the injury governs the treatment of the patient. He may be able to read aloud intelligently and also to write and yet be unable to carry on a coherent conversation owing to the difficulty of remembering the right word. It is at this stage that the therapist must try to get the patient to realize the value of relaxation in helping the memory to return.

How many of us fail to remember a name, try as we may, but when we have ceased to struggle with our memories the name flashes back to us, sometimes hours later. When dealing with an aphasic patient we should remember our own sense of frustration at such times and seek to apply the remedy we ourselves have tried to the patient.

No case of aphasia should be treated by a speech therapist without expert medical advice, as the nature and extent of this disorder is so varied and the association pathways so interwoven that it is necessary for a medical specialist to diagnose and suggest treatment. The speech therapist working under medical advice can safely introduce sense training and occupational therapy in an attempt to link up the faulty associations.

Miss Elsie Fogerty, whose work on Alexia (word blindness) is universally known, says:

Among the difficulties which have been met with in the treatment of children attending primary schools the greatest is the fact that they have lost step with their contemporaries in learning to read. The child whose word-blindness has been completely overcome is still in a measure in the same position as the normal child who has just learned to read. The ready vocabulary is small, sentence stress is uncertain, and there is no natural love of reading to induce constant voluntary practice. When these children return to the normal school class, where their contemporaries in age now have no further teaching in reading, they are often reported 'to read no better than they did before'. What is needed here is a special practice class for such cases, as it is difficult to keep them long enough at clinic to ensure complete fluency, and their own school teachers are better trained in the devices for teaching reading than the majority of clinicians.[1]

The disorder being due to a lesion in the brain between the visual and intellectual centre, it is necessary to approach the higher centres from a different angle; to do this the sense of touch should be developed. The child can be taught the meaning of symbols through touch and learns to connect the tactile impression with the written symbol. Sandpaper and block letters can be used for this purpose. See exercise, page 67.

[1] *Journal of Speech Disorders.*

CONGENITAL AUDITORY IMPERCEPTION

This is aphasia in the young child, but whereas the aphasic adult has spoken normally in the young child the speech faculty has not developed. The treatment should be on the same lines as that of Delayed Speech, i.e. sense-training, drawing block letters, etc. It is important that the child should have daily treatment if possible, but it must be of short duration as such a child tires very easily. It should be noted that the treatment is exhausting both to the patient and the therapist.

DISORDERS OF PHONATION

For all phonation disorders.

The nervous state of the patient should be treated through relaxation in order that all superimposed tension may be relieved before beginning exercises for the re-education of the voice. When the muscles of the throat are in the requisite condition, exercises for pure tone may be given with the utmost care, beginning with humming exercises on the 'M' sound.

FUNCTIONAL NASALIZATION (RHINOPHONIA)

Owing to insufficient movement of the velum, the nasal passage remains open. In order to correct this it is necessary to stimulate the movements of the soft palate; exercises for flexibility of the tongue and soft palate should be given, also for breath and voice direction. See pages 64 and 65.

DYSARTHRIA

DEAFNESS

It is essential to discover whether there is any deafness in a child suffering from a speech defect, as this disorder, however slight, may affect speech, and, in any case, causes nervous tension. The hearing of the child should be thoroughly tested before any treatment is undertaken. The speech of children suffering from total or severe deafness should only be treated by those who have undergone a specialized training.

Many of the children in the Special Schools for the Deaf are almost totally deaf and their speech is entirely learnt by lip reading. It is noticeable that the children talk freely to visitors, and have no difficulty in understanding their everyday speech.

The voice of the congenital deaf mute has a peculiar timbre and intonation, no matter how well he has been taught lip reading and articulation; on the other hand, the child who has become deaf after having heard for some time may retain a voice which is practically normal.

A further difficulty in deaf speech is the lack of inflexion and proper accentuation of the word; children of quick intelligence benefit from the excellent teaching that is being given in an endeavour to overcome this stupendous difficulty, but it is feared that children of slower intelligence often lose any ground that they have gained in this direction after leaving school.

As is well known, there is some difference of opinion as to the value and expediency of using the sign language. One of the most expert teachers of the deaf, although realizing the importance of oral teaching, does not deprecate the use of signs. At the 4th International Games for the Deaf, held in London in 1935, it was amazing to notice the extraordinary silence among thousands of people, most of whom were deaf. There were at least fourteen different nations competing and all seemed able to communicate with one another by means of the sign language. The doctor in charge, although not an expert in either form of communication, was able to make himself understood by signs to the various casualties that came under his care on the Sports Ground.

It is necessary that young children should learn to lip read and have oral teaching; at the same time the importance of sign language cannot be under-estimated. During recent years finger spelling has become unpopular, but, undoubtedly, it helps to increase vocabulary; this knowledge of words increases the interest, giving a broader outlook and another means of communication.

CLEFT PALATE AND KINDRED DISORDERS

In many cases the patient suffers from a triple handicap; the present discomfort following the pain and shock of the operation, the speech difficulty and a sense of inadequacy all combine to give the child a feeling of inferiority. In addition to the treatment for the organic defect it is essential that the child should be encouraged to develop any talent that he may possess to help the readjustment of his personality. If psychological guidance is not given the child may blindly compensate for his condition and a deeper psychological upset may result.

A girl of 15, suffering from a cleft palate, came to a Centre for Stammerers from a Training Home. In this case there was a great deal of superimposed tension in addition to the organic defeat; she had been abandoned by her mother in infancy—a fact which she attributed to her physical handicap. The Secretary of the Home took a personal interest in her and came to see us several times. Everything was done to facilitate the work, and arrangements were made to keep her in the Home for another year in order to enable her to improve her speech and adjust herself psychologically. She was in a very hysterical state when she came and was inclined to weep when her throat was examined. Soon, however, her confidence was gained, she learned to relax and joined happily in the games with the other children. Stammerers are usually sympathetic, and no surprise was shown at her nasal tone and cleft palate speech. At the end of a year she was satisfactorily placed in domestic service at the seaside; a year or so later she wrote saying that her speech had improved so much that many people had told her that they did not know that she had a cleft palate.

It is important that flexibility of the muscles affected by the operation should be induced. It is often desirable to begin with lip exercises, as even where there is no hare-lip the lips are frequently stiff through lack of use. The child probably has had many months of pain and discomfort, he had avoided using not only the affected muscles, but those which he feels may be affected; he therefore attempts to make all his sounds in the throat, thereby avoiding the pain of using the muscles of the tip of the tongue and the lips. The fine adjustments needed for the dental and liquid consonants cause a muscular movement of the tongue which exercises the whole of it; if the child fails to use his tongue there will be a lack of flexibility in the whole organ.

Where the lip muscles are particularly stiff, it is helpful to massage them with olive oil or cream before beginning treatment. The child will find it amusing to imitate a rabbit eating, smile and pout, and later attempt to whistle. The tongue exercises, which are fully described in Chapter V, may then be given, with exercises for breath direction and voice control.

For paresis of the velum and kindred disorders similar treatment may be given.

JAW DEFECTS AND DENTAL IRREGULARITIES

Dental treatment should be given as soon as possible. At the same time treatment should be undertaken by the therapist. Exercises for loosening the jaw and the muscles of the tongue are necessary, in conjunction with treatment for the sounds affected. See pages 58 and 59.

We have endeavoured to outline a general course of treatment for the commoner disorders of speech; but the co-operation of the patient is of the first importance, and we are convinced that a great deal of the therapist's success depends upon the power to inspire a wish in the patient to be cured.

When one of us was a student, she was asked how she would cure a faulty sound; she wrote, as she thought, a perfect description of the method to be used, ending with the words, 'The child would then produce the correct sound.' Professor Ripman wrote against it, '*Would* the child?' The truth of this remark has been proved times without number; in spite of the superior knowledge of the therapist, the child knows best and continues to produce his sounds as his fancy dictates.

CHAPTER IV

Psychogenic Disorders : Their Symptoms and Treatment

And Moses said unto the Lord, 'O my Lord, I am not eloquent
—but I am slow of speech, and of a slow tongue.'

THE disorders in this chapter, although affecting
speech, are not due to any functional or organic cause
but to some disturbance of the nervous system.

STAMMERING

The chief nervous disturbance affecting speech.

In the past many people tried to differentiate between
stuttering and stammering by saying that:

(a) Stuttering was a physical and stammering a
psychological defect.

(b) Stuttering was a rapid repetition of any one
sound (c-c-cat) and stammering an inability to
produce voice.

(c) Stuttering was a halt on consonants and stammering a halt on vowels.

Since it may be said that no two patients exhibit a
precisely similar stammer, each individual's particular
form, on this basis, would require a label of its own.

It is not advisable to differentiate between the terms,
and 'stammering' is preferable as representing all forms

of this disorder. In English literature 'stammering' has been used for 500 years, whereas 'stuttering' is low German and has only been in use for the past 100 years.
    Adler tells us:

Just as most diseases depend upon some constitutional organic anomaly, and a physical attempt to compensate for an inferior organ, so in the psychic field an inferior organ may give rise to an unconscious feeling of psychic inferiority and to compensatory mental mechanism.

According to this theory, neuroses and psychoses are the results of unsuccessful compensation; anxiety is an outstanding and common expression of the failure to compensate for some defect; and stammering is frequently a feature of an anxiety neurosis. Instances of psychic compensation are seen in the assumed self-assertion of the timid, one type indulging in over-dressing and vulgar ostentation, while another assumes a loud voice and a boastful manner. Defiance and resentment against authority, or a general 'naughtiness', are often symptoms of this same inferiority sense, symptoms in which the victim pretends to glory while inwardly he is miserably aware of failure. In fact, these are defence reactions.
    It is often said of stammerers that they push themselves forward; that they positively seek opportunities for speaking; and even that they do not mind stammering. If we might only enter the minds of these sufferers for a few hours and understand what they are really feeling under this apparent bluff, we should then realize to some small extent the martyrdom which they endure ceaselessly; a martyrdom aggravated by a constant sense of failure in spite of their most gallant efforts. 'They often disguise, under an air of indifference and tranquillity, the anguish of their hearts at their miserable infirmity.' So writes Forshaw, and a young man once

said, 'I often feel I would like to go somewhere right away and lose myself.'

Wendell Johnson, in his book *Because I Stutter*, gives a living and a moving description of the trials, hopes and fears of a stammerer. The following extract is typical:

Stuttering is a mental distraction and a physical drain on the energies of the individual. It interferes with his work in a school especially, not only because it forces him to think of himself constantly as being something of an exile, but also because the process of stuttering makes him, in the moment of stuttering, far less capable of carrying on the thought process than he otherwise would be ;—— Stuttering is a constant mental and physical pain, and although the stutterer learns, in time, to regard this pain nonchalantly, it remains important and can never be wholly disregarded.

The parents of a young child, especially when a first child is in question, are naturally immensely thrilled with his first utterances. But they seldom realize the tremendous expenditure of nervous energy required to learn new sounds. While in the meaningless babble stage the sounds produced present no difficulty, but as soon as intention appears, great concentration is required to ensure correct co-ordination. Everyone must have noticed the absorbed interest with which a child will watch and listen to a new sound combination; a word is repeated several times, he moves his lips and tongue in imitation at first, and finally produces, as nearly as he can, what he has seen and heard. If parents understood the amount of concentrated work required, they would be less inclined to force the child, and would allow him to develop this new talent at his own pace. It is a great temptation to show off the child to friends and relations, to prove his superiority to all other children by making him go through his linguistic paces, but it is a temptation that should be resisted. We should be very patient with the early attempts at speech. The critical adult who insists upon repetition of difficult sounds with 'Say it again, dear,' may very easily make the child speech-conscious and be the means of fixing a faulty speech sound or of inducing hesitation that may grow into a stammer.

At home, the mother can do much more than is generally realized to prevent stammering at its inception. Unfortunately, she is, more often than not, instrumental in fixing the trouble by making too much of the purely physiological stammer with which so many young children begin speech. When a baby is learning to walk he has many a fall before he acquires the co-ordination and control necessary for movement in the desired direction, and at the desired rate of progress. Learning to talk presents the same problem in a much more complicated form. The mechanism used in talking requires infinitely finer and more delicate adjustment than that used in walking.

At the initial stage of speech development, the mental process is in advance of the powers of muscular control, and the resulting lack of muscular co-ordination often produces a temporary stammer. If the child is worried and nervous during this period of adjustment, he will become conscious of his speech and of the difficulties surrounding its acquisition, and at once the second stage is reached—that of fear or dread of speech—unconscious probably, but none the less potent. Too much attention to the initial difficulties and constant correction or ridicule are usually the cause of this second stage, for which the parents are responsible, either applying the 'remedy' themselves or by allowing others to do so.

The method of treatment to be followed should be

relaxation and personality adjustment. This means the treatment of the stammerer and not of the stammer; in other words, concentration on the cause and not on the symptom. This appears to us to be the only satisfactory way to help the sufferer to recover mental and nervous poise without increasing his difficulties. The aim should be to distract the stammerer's attention from speech rather than to emphasize what is already an obsession. Methods that draw attention to the symptom rather than the cause often tend to aggravate the symptom.

It has been found beneficial to treat stammerers in groups. The stammerer is very often an introvert and his association with other sufferers makes him realize that his sense of isolation is exaggerated. The stammerer always feels that he is 'different' and does not realize that this sense of difference is common to all mankind. He finds, by working with others, that his difficulties are not unique, and the realization brings courage, confidence and a sense of comradeship. This change of outlook is often apparent shortly after treatment has begun.

All writers on this subject agree that there is a physical tension which varies according to the degree of the defect. Before any psychological adjustment can take place this tension must be relieved by relaxation. All attempts of the stammerer at speech are accompanied by over expenditure of energy; over expenditure in any physical action will cause faulty balance resulting in disco-ordinated movement. It is only necessary to watch a number of boys throwing a cricket ball to realize the truth of this statement.

The waste of nervous energy takes its physical toll and the patient, endeavouring to overcome this feeling of exhaustion, expends more nervous energy, and thus a vicious circle is formed.

A class of stammerers was asked to draw or write their ideas on the year, the therapist wanted to discover their powers of visualization; no mention of relaxation was made by her, but a boy of 13 wrote:

> I used to regard a year as one long period of dreary existence, dotted here and there with bright things that I used to say or do. School was utterly miserable, as my classmates were small boys of no feeling whatever. I used to hate to go on errands for my Mother, I tried to avoid it as often as I could, although I now see how foolish it was. But now my mind seems more clear. My outlook on my future life more happier. I enjoy seeing how (much) better I speak when I relax.

The first duty towards a stammerer, then, is to help to relieve the mental strain under which he lives, to tell him that by practising deliberate muscular relaxation he will gradually acquire greater ease of mind, which will, in turn, restore self-confidence, self-respect, and will, by degrees, eliminate the fear of speech. This also brings about a reconditioning and control of the neuro-muscular system.

The basis of all treatment for stammerers, whether individually or in groups, should be relaxation. It is impossible to insist too strongly upon this point. The curative value of relaxation is, unfortunately, not as yet sufficiently realized. It looks deceptively simple, but the true technique can be extremely elusive, and can be successfully imparted only by those who have themselves been through the whole process and who can themselves relax.

It is not only the stammer itself that derives benefit from relaxation; in fact, it is often the last symptom to yield to treatment. In the earlier stages of practice the patient usually shows improvement in general health; he finds himself able to face life more confidently; he worries less over trifles. Children very often show a marked improvement in school work or in games, with the gradual increase of confidence, concentration and co-ordination. It is remarkable, too, how they will lose the habit of enuresis, which has perhaps been chronic for years; some children have been known to cease the habit after the first week of attending a centre for stammerers. Similarly, headaches, constipation, nervous debility and kindred disorders will disappear under the influence of curative relaxation.[1]

The question of whole-time as opposed to part-time treatment for stammerers is one that is sometimes raised. It has been found that excellent results accrue where the children attend a centre twice weekly. The child's normal routine is hardly disturbed, and he is not made to feel that he is different from his fellows. Moreover, where reorganization of the nervous system is in progress, it is found that greater advance is made in the intervals than during the actual time of instruction, stimulation is far more effective if intermittent than if constant. Travelling to and from the Centre by tram or omnibus is often a decided help in restoring confidence to a hitherto timid child.

Whole-time treatment, on the other hand, tends to separate the individual too much from his fellows. It provides him with the ideal environment instead of helping him to adjust himself to, and to deal with, the existing home conditions. The result of this type of treatment is too often: 'I was perfectly all right while I was away, but as soon as I came home I found myself stammering again.'

[1] Cf. *Relaxation in Everyday Life*, Boome and Richardson.

5

APHTHONGIA

A condition in which the attempt to speak sets up severe spasms in the muscles of articulation, chiefly in the tongue. Nothing is known of the pathology; it may be akin to myotonia, tetany or occupation.[1] This condition may be similar to nervous lisping.

NEUROTIC SIGMATISM

If a lisper is made to feel speech-conscious through nagging or ridicule, the purely mechanical difficulty may become 'fixed' and a nervous inhibition is superimposed showing itself in an uncontrolled spasm on the sound affected. Both the stammerer and the neurotic lisper show excessive muscular tension; in the stammerer it is spasmodic, in the neurotic lisper constant. In a severe form the patient's mouth is often drawn sideways and the effect appears like that of a paralysis.

VOLUNTARY MUTISM

This condition sometimes occurs after either a mental or physical shock; it may be regarded as a form of aphasia. It is an hysterical condition and should be treated by relaxation and personality adjustment.

All defects of articulation, phonation and disorders of the language function may become psychological through wrong treatment. The child feels a sense of isolation which he may not understand but which gives him a severe sense of inadequacy. This sense may deepen as he grows older, affecting his whole personality, and that which started as a mechanical difficulty becomes a serious disturbance.

[1] James Collier.

CHAPTER V

Exercises for Relaxation and Disorders of Speech

A merry heart is better than a medicine,
But a broken spirit dryeth up the bones.

PROVERBS

IT is important that the whole personality of the patient should be considered in dealing with any form of speech disorder. The defect is so often the outward symptom of a much deeper disturbance; the patient, being highly sensitive over the disability, will often hide it by inaudibility or quick, hurried speech. Both these forms of speech are due to overanxiety which causes general or particular stiffening, giving both a sense of physical discomfort and of mental strain. Thus a vicious circle is formed, the mental anxiety causes physical tension, which in its turn wastes nervous energy, and this waste reacts again deleteriously on the mind.

It has been noticed that in a number of cases children suffering from functional speech defects have very little sense of general rhythmic movement or of their ability to make delicate co-ordinated movements of the hands and feet. They feel that the tongue is an unruly member over which they seem to have little control, and this local feeling of inadequacy often appears to extend to other movements of the body. When these children find

that they are able to do amusing exercises correctly
with their fingers a feeling of confidence is inspired
which goes a long way to remove the first obstacle to
improved speech.

The patient must become aware of the difference
between normal muscular tension and hypertension,
which is not only a waste of energy but a definite
hindrance to muscular action. In order to obtain this
awareness it is often necessary for the patient to learn
to relax muscle by muscle, and we find it helpful to
achieve this relaxation through the medium of muscular
movements.

In these preliminary exercises for relaxation, the
patient should be encouraged to use definite conscious
thought, in order to realize the sensations of the action
and to notice the difference in feeling between an easy
and a tense movement. It is important that the poise
of the body should be correct before any exercises are
attempted. The weight of the body should be evenly
balanced over the arch of the foot with a tendency to
keep the weight forward. This position eliminates any
possible chance of hypertension in the knee muscles
which upsets the perfect balance of the spine, neck and
head.

A Colonel once told his men that if they kept the
weight of the body on the ball of the foot they need
have no fear of fainting on parade. It is interesting to
note that none of his men ever fell out, however long
they were required to stand. It is not always realized
that it is possible to be 'at attention' and yet relaxed.

When the patient has gone through a series of muscular movements and has gained a feeling of general
loosening he is ready to relax. He should then lie down

flat on his back in as comfortable a position as possible; the hands lightly clasped with the fingers interlocked, and the feet crossed. He should close his eyes and try to relax the body by conscious thought. As the muscles relax there is a corresponding feeling of ease in all the organs of the body which shows itself in the ease and depth of the breathing, and a general feeling of warmth throughout the body. When the physical relaxation is complete the patient obtains a sense of mental ease; and after a period of relaxation is conscious of renewed nervous energy and a general sense of well-being.

We hope that the following exercises may be of some help to those who are dealing with disorders of speech.

RELAXATION

The basis of all movement is relaxation

PRELIMINARY EXERCISES TO RELAXATION

I. HEAD AND NECK EXERCISES (STANDING OR SITTING)

(a) Let the front neck muscles relax completely, so that the chin falls as far forward as possible; lift the head slowly, feeling the sensation in the back of the neck until the chin is in a level position. Then let the head fall slowly backwards so that the front throat muscles are stretched and the back of the neck is relaxed. It is most important that there be no suggestion of 'double chin' when the head falls forward, as this means the throat muscles are not relaxed.

(b) Turn the head from side to side, keeping the shoulders still and the poise of the body correct.

(c) Make a complete circle, rolling the head from left to right with the neck muscles relaxed and the chin forward.

These exercises should be repeated two or three times only, as they are rather tiring. If a collar is worn, it should be opened.

2. SHOULDER, ARM AND HAND MOVEMENTS

(a) *Shoulder Rolling Leading to Shoulder Swing*

With the arms hanging loosely at the sides roll the shoulders gently from front to back feeling the gradual increase in sensation extending through the entire arm. As the roll of the shoulders increases the arms describe a wider and wider circle, the weight of the downward movement causing the swing to increase and the arms to move of their own volition, ultimately leaving the sides and making the fullest extension above the head.

It is important that there should be no tension in the elbows, and that the shoulder movement should be increased at an even rate. This exercise must never be given starting from back to front.

(b) *Elbow Circling*

(i) *Downward Circle.* Extend the arms to shoulder level, palms facing downwards, describe a circle from the elbow downwards keeping the hands in a neutral position until the end of the movement, they will then be palm upwards; turn the elbow and repeat the exercise.

(ii) *Upward Circle.* Repeat the exercise, beginning with the palm upwards. The shoulders must never be raised beyond their natural level. It is important that the elbows should make a complete turn.

(c) *Wrist Circling*

Turn the wrists outward and inward making as big circles as possible. The fingers should be extended.

(d) *Wrist Dropping and Extending*

(e) *Finger Exercises*

    (i) Bend the fingers to touch the mount of the fingers and open.

    (ii) Close and open the whole hand with the fingers bent.

    (iii) Finger spreading.

        (a) Fingers opening and shutting, in unison.

> (*b*) Fingers opening and shutting separately, beginning with the thumb and first finger.

It is important to notice that the middle finger remains stationary, the first and third fingers move away from it.

(iv) Snake hands leading to arm movements.

> (*a*) Place the palms of the hands together, press the wrists, mounts of hands and finger tips until the fingers are horizontal, counting, '1, 2, 3 and away'.
>
> (*b*) Repeat the exercise with the palms apart and facing outwards, imagining the sensation of 'pushing' the air.
>
> (*c*) Repeat until the whole arm is moving in a snake-like manner. These finger exercises sometimes cause difficulty owing to the tendency to use too much energy; it is important that children should be encouraged to *feel* movements as they are practising them. There are many conjuring exercises for flexibility of the fingers which are helpful and amusing.

3. BODY MOVEMENTS FOR RELAXATION OF ABDOMINAL AND BACK MUSCLES

(i) Let the whole body drop forward, feet together and knees straight, trying to relax the upper part of the body, and noticing especially the head, neck and arms. When the relaxed body is as far forward as possible, a general stretching movement should take place in an attempt to touch the toes. This exercise may be varied by substituting a side swing for the stretching movement.

(ii) Stand in a good position, let the head fall back until the eyes are looking at the ceiling and then stretch the chest, shoulder and abdominal muscles upwards. The sensation will extend to the thighs and knees.

It is unnecessary to attempt an acrobatic feat, only the slightest backward bend is required.

(iii) Raise the arms sideways to shoulder level, turn the

body to right and left, keeping the hips in a stationary position.

4. SWIMMING EXERCISES

The difference in power in the first two movements should be noticed.

(*a*) With the palms of the hands together in front of the chest the arms shoot forward in a strong movement.

(*b*) The hands turn outwards to sweep the water and the power increases to its fullest extent.

(*c*) The hands and arms are brought back into a relaxed position.

The various swimming strokes can all be practised in this way, and the leg movements can also be attempted.

5. LEG EXERCISES

(*i*) *Leg Swinging*

Stand on one leg and swing the other backwards and forwards from the hip. The knee should be straight but relaxed.

(*ii*) *Knee Swinging*

Lift the thigh at right angles to the body, clasp the hands under the knee and swing the lower part of the leg. The arms should feel the weight of the thigh, but the elbows should on no account be tense as this will upset the balance. If the thigh is not at right angles there will also be lack of balance. When the knee is swinging, the ankle and foot should be in a relaxed position.

(*iii*) *Heel Raising and Knee Bending*

(*iv*) *Foot Movements*

      (*a*) Tiptoe exercises.

      (*b*) Heel and toe exercises.

      (*c*) Pointing and stepping exercises.

Any of the exercises taught in Greek dancing can be used.

To enable the patient to realize the value and universal use of relaxation it is often helpful to take as a simile the actions of an animal, especially of the cat family, before sleeping. A cat stretches every muscle of its body as a preparation for sleep, and human beings would do well to watch and imitate 'the harmless necessary cat'. Young children will enjoy imitating these stretching movements.

RELAXATION

1. Lie on the back in as comfortable a position as possible, preferably with the head on a cushion, the hands lightly clasped across the body with the fingers interlocked and the feet crossed.

2. Close the eyes and think of a feeling of ease. The patient should try to think through and loosen the whole body in a definite order.

If there have been any preliminary exercises it is often helpful to form a mental picture of the muscular action and the state of the body on its cessation. This mental picture induces the power of concentration on tranquillity; the will is used to relax the body, the body thus released from expenditure of superfluous energy reacts on to the mind and gives the patient that complete sense of mental and physical peace.

EXERCISES FOR CO-ORDINATED MOVEMENT WITH SPEECH

1. Speak the clock round, marking the quarters, half-hours and hours by clapping the left hand on the palm of the right hand. Repeat this exercise standing, with a swing of both arms to mark the beat. The arms should be lifted as far as possible above the right shoulder with the weight on the right leg; the left leg being relaxed and the heel slightly raised. Swing the arms and body to the left, changing the weight on to the left foot. The eyes follow the hands during the swing, thus giving an easy movement of the neck and head.

2. In class work, when it is sometimes necessary for children to form two lines, the following exercise is useful for concentration and co-ordination. The therapist says

'Step one, two', the child repeats the words during the movement, taking the first step as he says 'step', the second on 'one', and finishes the movement by closing his feet on 'two'. The second child says 'Step one, two, three', the third child goes back to 'step one, two', and this continues until two lines are formed.

3. Let the children march round the room marking the third, fourth or fifth step by clapping.

This exercise may be varied by one child speaking a nursery rhyme, while another child is moving to the rhythm and the rest of the class clapping.

SPEECH EXERCISES
For flexibility of the articulatory organs

1. TONGUE
    (i) Put the tongue out, as far as possible, and in again, keeping it straight.
    (ii) Curl the tip of the tongue and try to touch the chin.
    (iii) Curl the tip of the tongue up and try to touch the nose.
    (iv) Touch the left cheek with the tip of the tongue.
    (v) Touch the right cheek with the tip of the tongue.
    (vi) Make a circular movement in front of and behind the teeth.
    (vii) Place the tip of the tongue behind lower teeth with the lips closed. Bring the blade of the tongue up and out as far as possible with the mouth open.
    (viii) Place the tip of the tongue behind the top teeth, and repeat the exercise.

2. LIP EXERCISES
    (i) Smile and pout alternately.
    (ii) Imitate a rabbit eating.
    (iii) Stretch the upper lip over the lower and return to normal position.

    (iv) Repeat with the lower lip over the upper lip.
    (v) Whistling.

3. JAW EXERCISES
    (i) Open mouth wide ('AH' position) and close.
    (ii) Wedge. Cut a triangular piece of cardboard about two inches wide. Hold it vertically between the finger and thumb, and with a rhythmic wrist movement place the apex between the teeth for the 'AH' sounds and away from the mouth for 'she'. The finger and thumb can be used instead of a wedge.

Sa	Ka	She	Fa	Ra
Ka	Ka	She	Fa	Ra
Ra	Ka	She	Fa	Ra
Da	Ka	She	Fa	Ra
Pa	Ka	She	Fa	Ra
Fa	Ka	She	Fa	Ra

The hand movement is most important in this exercise.

4. BREATHING EXERCISES
    (i) Single nostril breathing.
    (ii) Breathe in through the nose and out through the mouth.
    (iii) Breathe in and out through the nose with the mouth shut.
    (iv) Breathe in through the nose with the mouth open. The movement of the tongue closing the back of the mouth should be felt in this exercise.

Position for Breathing

    It is essential that the patient should either stand or sit in a good easy position. The hands should touch the sides of the chest lightly at the level of the sixth and seventh ribs, the tips of the fingers should be slightly curved inwards so that the nails are touching the chest, the wrists should relax forward. The hands should not be placed with the palms touching the chest as this causes strain in the wrist which is liable to extend into the rest of the arm.

5. VOWEL SHAPING

The tip of the tongue should not move from its position behind the lower teeth during this practice, and the lips should never be drawn back beyond their natural width in any vowel or diphthong sound.

(a) Main Vowels

Lips rounded.
- 'OO'—little finger between the teeth, the lips rounded closely over the finger ('o').
- 'OH'—the thumb between the teeth, and the lips rounded over it ('O').
- 'AW'—the first, second and third fingers forming a pyramid, and the lips rounded ('$\underset{\text{OO}}{\text{O}}$').

Lips neutral.
- 'AH'—the first and second fingers between the teeth at right angles to the jaw.
- 'AY'—the same position as for 'AH' but the tongue is slightly arched.
- 'EE'—the same position as for 'AH' with the tongue fully arched.

(b) Subordinate Vowels

- 'oo'—as in hood,
- 'o' —as in hot,
- 'u' —as in hut,
- 'a' —as in hat,
- 'e' —as in head,
- 'i' —as in hid.

Sentence for Practice. I hid my hat in a hut in the wood because my head was hot.

(c) Main Diphthongs.

- 'I'—formed by the subordinate vowels 'u' and 'i', not 'AH' and 'EE'.
- 'OW'—formed by the subordinate vowels 'u' and 'oo', not 'AH' and 'OO'.
- 'OI'—formed by 'AW' and 'i', not 'AW' and 'EE'.

Diphthong Practice.
> 'I.' u, u-u, u-u-i, I.
> 'OW.' u, u-u, u-u-oo, Owl.
> 'OI.' AW, AW-AW, AW-AW-i, Oil.

6. CONSONANT PRACTICE

POSITIONS FOR THE CONSONANTS

Breath Stops

In the consonants 'P.B.', 'T.D.', 'K.G.', the breath is stopped at some point in the mouth; when it is released the sound occurs. These sounds cause special difficulty at the end of a word owing to the extra energy required for their production.

> 'P' and 'B'. The lips are pressed lightly together, stopping the breath. On the opening of the lips the breath is released, producing the sound.

> 'T' and 'D'. The breath is stopped by the tip of the tongue touching the hard palate immediately behind the top teeth.

> 'K' and 'G'. The breath is stopped by the back of the tongue touching the hard palate.

Continuants

In these consonants the breath is obstructed at some point by the lips, tongue or teeth.

> 'F' and 'V'. The top teeth touch the lower lip and the breath passes through the confined space.

> 'TH' (voiced and unvoiced). The tip of the tongue is placed between the teeth, the sound is made as the tongue is drawn smartly back across the top teeth.

> 'S' and 'Z'. The sides of the tongue are raised, forming a narrow channel down the centre of the tongue, through which the breath passes. The tip of the tongue must touch either the top or lower teeth. In normal speech both these positions of the tongue tip are used according to the sound that precedes or follows it. In cases of cleft palate or 'strident S' the sound should be practised with the tongue tip behind

the lower teeth, but in the correction of interdental fricative substitution it has been found helpful to use the upper teeth position.

'SH' and 'ZE' (as in rouge). The lips are rounded and the sides of the tongue are raised as in 's', but their contact with the top teeth causes the channel to be widened, so that the breath is more diffused.

'L.' The sound is produced by the front of the tongue touching the hard palate immediately behind the top teeth, allowing the breath to pass between the sides of the tongue and teeth.

'R.' Southern English 'r'. The tongue is raised, the tip is curled back resting on the hard palate, the air passing between this narrow passage causes the friction necessary for the production of this sound. The position of the tongue is the same for the trilled and untrilled sound, but in the former the vibrations are more numerous.

SEMI-VOWELS 'w' and 'y'

These sounds are neither true vowels nor consonants, as in each case there is a slight interference with the flow of the breath.

'W.' The lips are shaped as in 'OO', but move inwards; this friction causes the sound.

'Y.' The tongue is arched as in 'EE', but the definite pressure of the sides of the tongue on the upper teeth almost causes a breath stop.

'CH.' This sound is combination of 't' and 'sh' and causes trouble as it is a breath stop followed by a continuant.

NASAL CONSONANTS

'M.' 'N.' 'NG.'

'M.' The lips are closed lightly, the tip of the tongue touching the lower teeth and the breath passes out through the nose.

'N.' The blade of the tongue touches the teeth ridge and the breath passes through the nose.

'NG.' In this sound the back of the tongue and the soft
palate are approximated and the breath passes out
through the nose.

7. VOWEL AND CONSONANT PRACTICE

(i) *Vowels and Consonants*

Oot	oht	awt	aht	ayt	eet
Ood	ohd	awd	ahd	ayd	eed
Oop	ohp	awp	ahp	ayp	eep
Oob	ohb	awb	ahb	ayb	eeb
oof	ohf	awf	ahf	ayf	eef
Oov	ohv	awv	ahv	ayv	eev
Ook	ohk	awk	ahk	ayk	eek
Oog	ohg	awg	ahg	ayg	eeg

('g' is hard.)

Oos	ohs	aws	ahs	ays	ees
Ooz	ohz	awz	ahz	ayz	eez
Oosh	ohsh	awsh	ahsh	aysh	eesh
Ooge	ohge	awge	ahge	ayge	eege

('ge' *as in* 'rouge'.)

Ooch	ohch	awch	ahch	aych	eech

('ch' *as in* 'each'.)

Ooj	ohj	awj	ahj	ayj	eej

('j' *as in* 'judge'.)

Oost	ohst	awst	ahst	ayst	eest
Oosts	ohsts	awsts	ahsts	aysts	eests
Ooth	ohth	awth	ahth	ayth	eeth
Ooths	ohths	awths	ahths	ayths	eeths
Oodth	ohdth	awdth	ahdth	aydth	eedth
Oodths	ohdths	awdths	ahdths	aydths	eedths
Oom	ohm	awm	ahm	aym	eem
Oon	ohn	awn	ahn	ayn	een

All practice should be given to some definite rhythm,
which can be marked by the arms, hands, wrists or fingers.
All difficult sounds should be practised in triple rhythm.

(ii) ttt, ttt, ttt, town, marking the beat by tapping one
finger of the left hand on the right hand.

(iii) Compound Sounds. Practice each sound separately, at first slowly—gradually increasing the pace.

'CH.' Example: 'T'...................'Sh'.
'T'...............'Sh'.
'T'...........'Sh'.
'T'........'Sh'.
'T'....'Sh'.
'Tsh.' = Church.

'PL.'   'P'...................'L'.
'P'...............'L'.
'P'...........'L'.
'P'........'L'.
'PL.' = Please.

'L' preceded by a breath stop causes considerable difficulty.

8. EXERCISES FOR SOFT PALATE
    (i) Breathing exercises.
    (ii) Blowing exercises.
    (iii) Nasal consonant practice.
    (iv) Yawning.

In cases of cleft palate, post adenoid speech and all types of excessive nasality it will be found helpful to practise yawning before the vowel sounds.

Blowing exercises are a most important part of the treatment in cleft palate and kindred disorders and have to be practised over so long a period that the child's interest may flag. In order to keep alive the interest it is often necessary to devise exercises wherein the imagination may play a large part; for instance, in blow football the children like to feel that they are representatives of a famous football team.

Blowing exercises, as:
    (i) Blow football. This can be played with sticks of macaroni and a ping-pong ball or feather on a table with a smooth surface; or with a ping-pong ball on a bowl of water.

(ii) Paper-boat races.
(iii) Hum and blow on a comb covered with tissue-paper.
(iv) Blowing a penny whistle or flute.
(v) Blowing balloons.

NASAL CONSONANT PRACTICE

(*i*) *Practice*
    (*a*) Close the lips lightly and hum the sound, feeling the vibration on the lips.
    (*b*) Pluck the lips with the finger. If the production is correct there should be a twanging sound. If the tongue is drawn back this sound will not be heard.

(*ii*) '*N*' *Practice*
    Hum the sound, feel the vibration by touching the nostrils lightly with the fingers.

(*iii*) '*NG*' *Practice*
    (*a*) Breathe in through the nose with the mouth open on the sound 'NG', and out of the mouth on 'AH', silently.
    (*b*) Repeat the exercise in a whisper.
    (*c*) Repeat on a singing note.
    (*d*) Repeat the words: Ding-dong, Sing-song, Ping-pong, Tongue-tongue, using an arm movement to represent bell-ringing. This exercise can be used as a refrain in nursery rhymes about bells.

Example
    Merry go the bells, and merry do they ring,
    Ding-dong, Sing-song, Ping-pong, Tongue-tongue,
    Merry was myself, and merry did I sing;
    With a merry ding-dong, ding-a-ling-dee
    And a merry sing-song merry let us be!
    Ding-dong, Sing-song, Ping-pong, Tongue-tongue.

Simple Sentences for Practice
    'A.' Arthur aimed his arrow at the apple.
    'B.' Billy bought bananas for breakfast.
    'C.' Centipedes are circling in the centre of the ceiling.

6

'D.' Derrick drove ducks and drakes down the dirty ditch.

'E.' Eva endeavours to eat eleven enormous eggs.

'F.' Forty-four foxes foraged in the forest.

'G.' Gordon goes into the garden to gather green goose-
berries.

'H.' Hannah holds a heavy hammer in her hand.

'I.' Ivan was isolated by the ice on the Isis.

'J.' Jimmy enjoyed jam and jelly from Jamaica.

'K.' Kenneth kicked the kitchen kettle.

'L.' Lionel looked at the lazy lion lying among the lilies.

'M.' Mother made marsh mallows, meringues and mince
meat.

'N.' Nelly noticed nine nightingales at the New Inn.

'O.' Obadiah wrote an ode to the old oak in Ohio.

'P.' Peter put the pepper on his plate.

'Q.' Queenie quits the quaint quarry with quarts of
quinces.

'R.' Reggie ran right round the red rock.

'S.' Sarah saw seven silver sixpences shining on the
sideboard.

'T.' Tommy took ten tiny tin-tacks.

'U.' Una and the unicorn are under the umbrella.

'V.' Vera is very vain of her violet velvet.

'W.' Willy wears worsted woollens in the winter.

'X.' The examiners set excellent exercises for the Ex-
mouth examination.

'Y.' Yolande yawned at the Yuletide yodelling yesterday.

'Z.' Zoe's zebra zigzagged zealously at the Zanzibar Zoo.

'SH.' Sheila shines Shirley's shabby shoes.

'CH.' Charley churns cheerfully chewing cherries.

'TH.' There are thirty-three thrushes in that thicket.

'PL.' The Ploughman and the plumber plotted to plaster
the Plymouth-plate.

'PR.' Prunella presented primroses to the princess.

'BL.' The blizzard blackens the bloom of the blossom.

'CL.' Clara clamoured for clean clothes.

'GL.' The glowworm glistened gloriously in the gloaming.

'ST.' Stanley stood on the steps of the station staring at the stars.

'SK.' The skilled skipper skimmed the skilley.

'SC.' Scott scanned the Scotch schooner for scallops.

'SL.' The slender sloop slipped slowly from the slips.

'SP.' The Spaniard spells speedily at the spelling-bee.

'SPR.' The sprite sprang sprily in the springtime.

'SQU.' The squeamish squirrel squatted in the square.

'STR.' Strephon strewed straw on the strawberries by the stream.

'SCR.' The scraggy scribe scribbled the screed in the scrub.

'SH-S.' The shepherd sings sylvan songs in the sunshine.

'SHR.' The shrew and the shrike shrieked in the shrub on Shrove Tuesday.

'SH-CH.' The shopper bought a cheap chopper at the shop to chop chips.

'TH-S.' Thelma sowed thorn trees, salsify and thistle-down.

'F-TH.' Forty thousand foresters fought fifty thousand thieves.

'ST.' Mr. West missed the last post to the coast.

'ND.' He found a pound in the sand by the bandstand.

'LD.' The child held the golden shield for the soldier.

'ST.' Mr. Lister and his sister roasted chestnuts at Easter.

'CT.' The Rector lectured in October on the picture of the octopus.

'TL.' The little bottle rattled in the metal scuttle.

EXERCISES FOR APHASIA [1]

(i) Relaxation.

(ii) Articulatory exercises as required.

(iii) Chewing and yawning.

(iv) Sense training exercises.

(v) Word blindness.

[1] *Journal of Speech Disorders*, by kind permission of Elsie Fogerty, C.B.E., L.R.A.M. See Appendix IV.

WORD BLINDNESS

1. The first exercise given is Blind Reading. Very solid wooden block letters are employed, the child standing with his back to the teacher, a letter is placed in his hand held behind the back. The name of the letter is then given and the peculiarities of the shape described. This is continued without any use of sight until all the letters can be named phonically and alphabetically: 'Its name is Bee, and it says Buh, &c.'

2. The process is repeated while the child draws a rough sign for the letter in the air with the forefinger.

3. The process is repeated, but after naming each letter the child looks at it and puts it down in front of him.

4. The child is now asked not to name the letter until after he has looked at it, and where this is not successfully done he returns to the blindfold feeling.

5. The child looks at the letter, names it and tests the correctness of his impression by feeling the letter.

6. Block-letter drawing is now introduced, and all the impressions are compared and used in haphazard order, e.g. look at it, draw it, name it, feel it, sound it.—Look at it, sound it, draw it, name it, feel it, &c., &c.

7. Very large printed letters are now employed, the child tracing them with his hand held by the teacher, naming them, looking at them, repeating the name.

8. The next stage—word reading—is difficult from the impossibility of obtaining good carved combinations of sounds or raised word blocks, but by this time words printed under as in ordinary reading books, have generally become fairly intelligible, and the order look, speak, copy, write, is found useful.

It should be noted that the first block-letter feeling is never given up, as it is obvious that this is the link which re-established connection between the visual impression and the word Motor-Memory.

9. Without giving up the general curative practice, an attempt is now made to teach the child reading in the ordinary way. It is here that the school-teacher's help is most valuable.

CHAPTER VI

The Speech of the Mentally Defective

He that shall be said to be a sot and idiot from his birth is such a person who cannot count or number twenty pence, nor tell who was his father or mother, nor how old he is, so as it may appear that he hath no understanding nor reason of what is to his profit or for his loss ; but if he hath sufficient understanding to know and understand his letters, or read by teaching or information, then it seems he is not an idiot.

An old legal definition of mental deficiency by L. C. J. HALE, *at the beginning of the seventeenth century.*

THE term Mental Deficiency is often used loosely to define all disorders of the mind from decay of normal intelligence through disease or old age to that of a mind without the innate power to develop. Thus the term Dementia and Amentia.

Tredgold says:

Mental defect occurring subsequently to mental development may be compared to a state of bankruptcy, and is more fittingly described as dementia (de, down from; mens, mind); whilst the person whose mind has never attained normal development may be looked upon as never having had a banking account, and this state is designated amentia (a, without; mens, mind).

For purposes of grading it has been found expedient to divide those suffering from mental defect into three groups.

1. Feeble minded.
2. Imbeciles.
3. Idiots.

These are again subdivided into High, Medium and Low grade. It is obvious that a great gulf exists between the High Grade Feeble minded and the Low Grade Idiot.

Aristotle described and posterity has accepted four different types of temperament.

1. Choleric—excitability great, and after effect great.
2. Sanguine—excitability great, and after effect small.
3. Phlegmatic—excitability small, and after effect small.
4. Melancholic—excitability small, and after effect great.

In normal people these emotions are controlled by civilization and environment; in the mentally defective child the emotions control the behaviour, he has neither the desire nor the power to conform to the accepted laws of society; he is anti-social and consequently his tendency is to destroy rather than to create.

In what way does the speech of the mentally defective child vary from that of the normal child? The first thing to be considered is what is good speech? It has been previously observed that it is the perfect co-ordination of sound, movement and understanding; if there is a fault in any of these the instrument will not play in tune, each of them must harmonize with the others for perfect utterance.

The higher we get in the intellectual world the more subtly modulated is the voice; this does not necessarily mean that the possessor of a great intellect is the possessor of a beautiful voice but that the thought behind the words controls the inflexion of the voice and by its modulation is the thought made clear. The alteration of pitch, of volume and of pace, the pauses between the words render the thought into coherent and beautiful speech.

The voice is the reflection of the mind, if the mind is flawed the reflection is dulled. The voice of the mentally deficient child shows this clearly; the low-grade child speaks in a dull monotonous voice with practically no change of pitch unless he is upset or excited; when this occurs the pitch may alter considerably, but it is comparable with the strumming of a child on the piano, he is incapable of discriminating between pleasant chords and discords.

The higher-grade children show much greater variety of pitch and in many cases their voices will pass muster for general use, but the finer shades are missing and the slightest emotion will affect the modulation.

Between these grades are found many types of voice, among which are the hoarse, harsh variety, which seems unable to produce a purely voiceless sound; its opposite, the nervous whispering voice, which reflects the lack of confidence in the child's mind; and the high-pitched voice of the emotionally unstable. The state of mind of the child is clearly indicated through the tone he produces. It was noticed that the temper of the children could be gauged by the singing of the hymn at Prayers. If anything had occurred to upset them, their singing was harsh and out of tune.

Mentally defective children often suffer from sense deprivation as well as lack of motor control.

> They have mouths, but they speak not;
> Eyes have they, but they see not;
> They have ears, but they hear not;

Noses have they, but they smell not;
They have hands, but they handle not;
Feet have they, but they walk not;
Neither speak they through their throat.

The mind of the normal child is built up through associations caused by sensations, the number and integrity of these determine the quality of his mind.

The brain of the newborn child consists of a gelatinoid substance, in which are embedded myriads of embryonic nerve cells; but these cells, or neuroblasts, are so immature that mind can hardly be said to have an existence. It is by means of incoming nervous vibrations transmitted through the peripheral organs and along the avenues of sensation that these neuroblasts derive their chief stimulus to growth, and consequently by which mental activity comes into being. The cerebral cells must, of course, possess an innate capacity to develop; indeed, it is a defeat of this capacity which constitutes the essential feature of amentia. But there is every reason to believe that not only is this stimulation from without vital to their development, but that ideation, judgment, reasoning, even will, are dependent upon the quantity and quality of the sensations received from the outside world. We may, indeed, say that sensations are the bricks out of which mind is built, and that in their absence the brain cells are incapable of producing a single idea. As in the newborn child, sensation may be present without reason, but reason cannot exist without sensation.[1]

Disorders of speech arise from defects of the Sensory, Intellectual and Motor Pathways.

SENSORY DEFECTS

(a) HEARING AND LISTENING. It is important to differentiate between true congenital or acquired deafness and inability to listen. Listening requires the use of the will to enable the mind to concentrate. Any form of concentrated attention is difficult to the ament and possibly listening is the most difficult of all, due, partly

[1] *Mental Deficiency*, Tredgold.

to the fact that sight and touch quickly distract his attention and, also, that his limited reasoning capacity fails to grasp the meaning of the sounds.

Although the mentally defective child has very little power of creating his own image pictures, he enjoys being helped to create, and delights to listen and repeat the natural sounds of birds, animals and insects. These children know the commoner types of animal life, either by sight or from pictures, and find great pleasure in repeating the sound, also, in many cases, in imitating the antics of the creature in question. All the pure vowel sounds can be taught in this way.

In order to avoid confusion in a mind already confused, it is most important that the child shall first have a clear mental picture before attempting an imitation.

In a class of low-grade children an experiment was made with a telephone game. The children had all seen and heard a telephone used. The class picked up an imaginary instrument, listened, and then gave an imaginary order for an exercise in movement or speech. The whole class then endeavoured to carry out the order given; if any mistake was made the class rang up the imaginary 'shop' and repeated the original order. This order and response were repeated until both were correct. It is essential that one idea only shall be given, and that it shall be within the capacity of the class to carry out.

(b) SEEING AND LOOKING. As in the case of hearing and listening, seeing is a physiological, looking a psychological, function. The mentally defective child may have adequate sight, but weak visual perception. This probably accounts for the great difficulty he has in learning to read. The use of pictures, small block letters made of wood or sandpaper, will enable the child to perceive the shape and thus visualize the words he is endeavouring to read.

If the mentally defective child can read it is helpful to him as it fosters a sense of adequacy and decreases the feeling of difference from normal children. These children are very proud of their prowess in this direction and take a delight in showing that they can read. If, however, reading can only be taught at too great a cost of nervous energy, the time would be better spent in learning some handicraft which would, in another form, alleviate this sense of inadequacy.

The Superintendent of a Certified Institution for the Mentally Defective had a special night school for reading. The patients attended voluntarily. Some of them could read a little, some hardly at all; the fact that the acquisition of reading would enable them to be allowed out on licence acted as a strong incentive. This teaching, in addition, gave them increased self-confidence and a greater social sense.

(c) TASTE. In many cases the sense of taste is defective. A mentally defective boy of 12 years (personally known to the authors) ate large portions of a door-mat with no ill results.

It has been suggested that the undeveloped sense of taste may have a bearing on the insensitiveness of the tongue in the matter of touch; this theory cannot yet be fully accepted as the speech work among mentally defective patients is at present only in the experimental stage.

INTELLECTUAL DEFECTS

The lack of power of understanding and visualizing words.

The normal child collects ideas through association

and creates mental pictures which may or may not be accurate, but which give him a clear idea of the words spoken; the defective child is almost entirely lacking in this gift of imagination, and can, as a rule, only understand what he has already seen. This lack of visualization is one of the chief causes of their inability to listen.

Speech Defects due to faults in the Intellectual Pathway:

(a) Delayed Speech. This condition in varying degrees is very often found among mentally defective children.

(b) Idioglossia, Echolalia and certain forms of Lalling may also be termed intellectual defects. These disorders have been fully described in a previous chapter.

MOTOR DEFECTS

The ament is an unfinished product and has many physioiogical difficulties in addition to the psychological. The high palatal arch and abnormal velum, so prevalent among these patients, causes special difficulties in speech.[1] The incidence of cleft palate is almost that of normal children, but owing to the mental

[1] 'Enlarged tonsils, adenoids, and nasal obstructions are far more common among defectives than among normal individuals of the same class. With these are often associated deafness and visual defects which, if not recognized and treated, add to the original deficiency the effects of partial sensory deprivation. Deformities of the palate are common, the main types being an unusually high and narrow V-shaped arch, or an unusual flatness. Wallis points out that much of the apparent arching of the palate in defectives is due to hypertrophy of submucous tissues, and not to arching of the bone. In his experience the broad, flat type is the more common. Cleft palate and hare-lip, though representing the persistence of foetal condition, are not regarded as stigmata of degeneration.'—*Mental Deficiency Practice*, Shrubsall and Williams.

condition, the patient is unable to concentrate sufficiently to improve at an even rate. The tongue is often
clumsy and appears to have no tip, the muscles insen-
sitive to the finer adjustments for articulation. In addition the jaws are often misshapen, narrow, overshot and
underhung. The consequent dental trouble makes an
additional difficulty with speech. Functional nasalizing
is also very common among the mentally defective.
When the development is arrested there is often a high
degree of indistinctness due to blurred tone. This condition is often spoken of as 'Mentally Defective Speech'.

In the speech treatment of defective children many
difficulties are encountered which do not arise among
normal children. The children are of so many types and
of such different grades that it is dangerous to generalize.
The psychotic child is excitable, overstimulated and
unstable; he is an egoist and his outlook on life often
entirely selfish. He has very little feeling of *esprit de corps*
and does not understand the team spirit. Occasionally
he will co-operate with other children in class exercises,
but his attention quickly wanders. When he is not the
centre of interest, his object appears to be iconoclastic,
he wishes to destroy the thing in which he feels he has
no part.

The lethargic child, on the other hand, gives little
trouble, but he is in constant need of stimulation; he
apparently lives in a world of his own and appears
unconscious of much that is happening around
him.

The higher- and middle-grade feeble-minded children
often show great unselfishness and in later years possess
a power of devotion and unselfishness which is not
always apparent in their more fortunate brothers and
sisters of normal intelligence.

Initiative is one of the most strongly marked characteristics of the normal child; he must do things for himself, his early efforts are not always crowned with success but he learns to discriminate by experience. He learns that coal is not a staple form of diet, but he also learns that legs are meant for walking and that the constant falls he endures in trying to walk are because he is not sufficiently experienced in the exercise. He knows that his kind are meant to walk on two legs and he practises until he is proficient and the action automatic. In the same way he practises all kinds of sounds with his mouth and tongue, providing himself with a strong foundation upon which to build his speech. He uses his lips and tongue and finds that by placing them in various positions they produce pleasant sounds; he practises and as he does so he gets the sensation of power over these organs and they obey him. He acquires the habit of correctly placing his sounds and his speech becomes his servant.

The mentally defective child is without this desire to be master of himself. Slowly his body acquires a certain proficiency of action, but the central force being imperfect there can be no real co-ordination. Faulty sensations have been previously mentioned and this insensitiveness appears in strange ways; often these children seem to feel little pain when they are hurt, they can eat things which would make a normal child ill for days, even perhaps kill him, yet they themselves may die from illnesses which the normal child hardly feels. The mentally deficient child has little stability, and this lack of responsibility underlies everything he does. If he is helped and looked after, he can often produce good work, but he cannot be left to initiate; he cannot plan his actions and carry them out.

As a baby, the higher-grade mental defective possibly made much the same sounds as his more fortunate brothers, also his inherited instincts probably led him along the right lines, but that lack of faith in himself gave him no impetus to practise in the way of the normal child. The child will master simple words easily enough and be able to carry on a conversation, but he will avoid any difficult combination whenever possible. In many cases these children cannot read and their knowledge of words is from ear alone, the sound has to pass through a faulty brain before it can be brought out in speech. The wonder is, not that the child makes a poor attempt at it, but that he achieves anything approaching the actual word.

The lower-grade child is in a still more unfortunate position for speech. He has, more often than not, little control over his limbs, his walk is awkward and his power over his hands is inadequate; also he gets easily tired. It may be argued that one of these children will sit for an hour or more doing some constructive work such as cross-stitch, and that, therefore, his powers of concentration are good; this fact only proves that the action is so simple that it quickly becomes a habit. The habit acquired, the action becomes automatic and his conscious brain is not required to operate; he is also able to see a quick return for his work and this gives him pleasure. It is not real concentration but apparent.

Now, what happens in speech? He is expected to produce sounds with a faulty instrument; the speech organs themselves may be formed correctly, there is usually no organic defect, but the child, as a baby, was able to make no use of those periods of practice and is now asked to put language on to an inadequate basis.

In addition to the lack of initiative and co-operation

the defective child has very little power of reasoning or ability to see beyond the present. He can be amused and interested up to a point, but beyond that he becomes confused and is not capable of concentration for any length of time. The neurotic type delights in destroying and will smash things from sheer joy. The teachers in the Special Schools endeavour to educate through sense training. As the child realizes his power of achievement, he knows the joy of creation which sublimates the destructive habit and slowly the behaviour improves.

If the treatment is on the right lines, the improvement in speech and behaviour should be parallel. Before attempting to teach the low-grade defective child to speak, he must be ready for speech, otherwise it is acquired at the expense of the development of another part of his personality. These cases will benefit by sense training and rhythmic exercises for general co-ordination leading up to speech.

The value of relaxation for all types of mentally defective children has been proved. In one hospital where the excitable neurotic children predominated it was found necessary to practise muscular relaxation for three months before it was possible to do any speech work. Difficulties were experienced at first, but after a time the children appreciated the quietness, and through the co-operation of the Headmistress and Staff, daily practice was carried out. At the end of that time the children were divided into groups for speech work, and the more serious cases of speech defect treated individually. Every group began the lesson by relaxing.

In the treatment of individual cases of speech defect, the error should be criticized and not the child; these children are easily discouraged but their ambition can be stimulated by praise. Never infer 'You are stupid, and therefore incapable of making the sound', but rather suggest 'What a poor sound for such a clever child to make'.

Interest can be aroused by the dramatization of nursery rhymes and co-ordinated exercises through the medium of mime. For all defects of the velum blowing games can be enjoyed. A ping-pong ball on a bowl of water is a very efficacious and exciting exercise, though liable to cause damage to clothing; a paper boat on a smooth surface is equally useful and certainly drier.

The high palatal arch and abnormal velum referred to previously partly accounts for the dull lifeless tone, blurred articulation and functional nasalizing so preva-lent among defective patients. This condition becomes more noticeable as the child approaches puberty.

The physiological and neurological changes which take place at this period often have a considerable effect on the physique and personality of the normal child, causing him self-consciousness over speech and be-haviour. Normally the mental and physical develop-ment is at an even rate, so that in due course these diffi-culties solve themselves and full maturity is reached. In the case of the mentally defective this normal course is not followed as the physical powers develop at a greater rate than the mental. The adult defective has often great physical strength but his mentality prevents him from reaching physical perfection.

The physical appearance of the higher-grade child often seems normal, the difference between his mental and actual age not being at great variance. The mental age of the adult rarely reaches 10, consequently the discrepancy between the mental and the physical appears greater as years go on. In the lower-grades this discrepancy shows itself in the clumsy awkward gait, shuffling feet and general lack of rhythm.[1]

Perfect poise is seen in the walk of the Eastern woman carrying her water-pot, the balance of the body must be so adjusted that the movement is from head to foot and foot to head. The head is erect, the hips swing easily, carrying the whole movement of the body down to the rhythmic action of the feet, which is heel, ball of the foot and toe. In the mentally defective this balance is lacking, the head is rarely poised, consequently the general appearance is round shouldered; the hip movement is poor and is replaced by that of the knees. There is little foot action, the patient seems to put it flat upon the ground and the result is an ungainly shuffle. The general impression is an unfinished product.

We have said that speech is man's highest achievement, but perhaps next to this is the power of transmitting thought without speech; the poise of the body can express the state of mind, the synchronization of thought and the finest of physical movements result in facial expression. The eyes are the windows of the psyche, and, in the normal, can communicate and

[1] 'In the mentally defective, there is often a vacancy or lack of expression in the countenance or a constant overaction of the frontal muscles, producing horizontal wrinkles in the forehead, a knitting of the eyebrows, or a constant and possibly a symmetrical grimacing whenever the subject attempts active thought. This waste of muscular effort is specially associated with mental inferiority and is often combined with subnormal tone. The lack of neuro-muscular balance and education is also shown by kypholordosis and by a dropping position of the extended arms. Delay in sitting up as well as in commencing to walk is characteristic of mental deficiency. The gait of defectives is often clumsy and shuffling, with a stiffness that at first sight suggests spasticity, their movements are slow and often their reflexes are sluggish.'— *Mental Deficiency Practice*, Shrubsall and Williams.

7

interpret thoughts without verbal speech. When the mind is impaired the facial expression can only convey primitive emotions and is incapable of interpreting anything but the simplest thought of others. The mental defective can understand expressions of pleasure and displeasure, but the finer adjustments of facial expression are lost. As speech is the highest form of expression, the result of a union of physical and intellectual movement, any flaw in the intellect will affect either the mechanical utterance or the inflexion of the voice.

'If language is ultimately the creation of the intellect, yet hardly less fundamentally is the intellect a creation of language.'

CHAPTER VII

The Difficult Child: His Inhibitions and Characteristics

Man is so formed that by dint of being told that he is a fool he believes it, and by dint of telling himself so makes himself believe it.

PASCAL

THE child with a speech disorder very often develops a sense of inadequacy. The best definition of the nervous child is that of Cameron, who called it 'the difficult child', and this does not really cover the whole subject.

The difficult child we know too well; eager, thin, pale, wasting his little body with the intense energy which he puts into the whole business of life, a bad sleeper, a notable refuser of food, often squinting or stammering, or incontinent of urine, especially subject to strange 'bouts' or 'turns' or 'attacks' as the mother calls them, marked by increase of pallor, by prostration, by a furred tongue, foul-smelling breath, constipation, irregular pyrexia, and so forth.[1]

Many of these children have little power of concentration owing to the constant waste of nervous energy; they are inattentive in school with the result that they get behind in their work. Some parents and teachers, with the intention of spurring a child on who is backward, will exaggerate his shortcomings to him in the hope that he will make greater efforts. It is sometimes

[1] H. C. Cameron.

83

also said that the child is mentally defective or will have to go to a special M.D. School. This is heard by the child's fellows, who are not always sympathetic, and they further add to the child's distress by saying that he is 'barmy', &c. The child gets more and more dispirited and gives himself up as hopeless unless something is done.

This sense of inferiority, although by no means confined to the nervous children, is one of the characteristics which they all share in common, and which is largely due—in a child at any rate—to environment. Constant fault-finding and discouragement can only be withstood by the strongest and most independent characters; the others are gradually worn down until, from doubting their ability to do well in any given direction, they become quite certain of their inability to do so.

If those in the child's immediate environment would only realize that awkwardness, clumsiness, gaucherie and similar traits are symptoms of nervous strain, and would try to find and remedy the cause, there would be fewer unhappy and maladjusted people in the world. Unfortunately, these symptoms are too often treated with ridicule or punishment, which, instead of correcting the trouble, only serve to increase it.

The most diligent search could hardly yield a better example of a nervous child than Charles Lamb, whether studied from the point of view of his neuropathic inheritance and environment, or from that of his personality and temperament. Fitzgerald's absorbing history reveals this in abundant detail.

Charles Lamb's father was in a state of doddering imbecility during his last years; a querulous old bore whose one object in life was cribbage. Charles, then a young man, hardly more than a boy, was frequently dragged from his evening meal and kept up late at night by his father's passion for the game, who would querulously say, 'If you won't play with me, you might as well not come home at all.' Charles says in a letter to Coleridge:

I get home at night o'erwearied, quite faint, and then to cards with my father, who will not let me enjoy a meal in peace; but I must conform to my situation. I hope I am, for the most part, not ungrateful.

Mrs. Lamb was an invalid, suffering from an infirmity, presumably of nervous origin, which deprived her of the use of her limbs. She had three children, of whom the oldest, John, was her favourite. This son was an overbearing individual; Proctor wrote of him:

I do not retain an agreeable impression of him; if not rude, he was sometimes, indeed generally, abrupt and unprepossessing in manner. He was assuredly deficient in that courtesy which usually springs from a mind at friendship with the world.

Mary, Charles' sister, ten years his senior, suffered from recurring attacks of insanity, during one of which she killed their mother.

Charles himself was, as a child, small for his age, physically delicate and, psychologically, almost morbidly sensitive and shy. He was also a stammerer. In spite of this he was popular at school, as is shown by a fellow scholar, Charles Le Grice, who wrote:

Lamb was an amiable, gentle boy, very sensible, and keenly observing, indulged by his school fellows and by his master on account of his infirmity of speech. His step was plantigrade, which made his walk slow and peculiar, adding to the staid appearance of his figure—his delicate frame and his difficulty of utterance which was increased by agitation, unfitted him from joining in any boisterous sport.

This 'difficulty of utterance' also prevented him from

gaining an exhibition and instead of going to the University when he left school, he became a clerk in the South Sea House, and later in the East India Company.

In his *Recollections of Christ's Hospital* Lamb wrote of the Blue Coat boy:

> Within his bounds he is all fire and play; but in the streets he steals along with all the self-concentration of a young monk. He is never known to mix with other boys; they are a sort of laity to him. All this proceeds, I have no doubt, from the continual consciousness which he carries about with him of the difference of his dress from that of the rest of the world.

Thus wrote he of the Christ's Hospital boy in general, but it would be hard to find a more apt description of Lamb himself, or one more typical of a stammerer, with his 'continual consciousness of difference', due to his infirmity of speech. Lamb gives us a further glimpse of his attitude towards life in his *Maria Howe*.

> They (his family) loved pleasures, and parties, and visiting, but as they found the tenor of my mind to be quite opposite, they gave themselves little trouble about me, but on such occasions left me to my choice, which was much oftener to stay at home, and indulge myself in my solitude, than join in their visits.

Lamb's intellectual powers were of the highest order and he had a lively sense of humour; his conversation, among friends, often sparkled with wit in spite of his disability. He was temperamentally volatile and excitable, easily uplifted and easily downcast, sensitive and emotional; and yet, like so many stammerers, he possessed an underlying strength of character. In Lamb's case this last quality manifested itself in his sympathetic tolerance towards his father and brother, and his undying devotion to his sister. From a letter to Coleridge, written after the tragedy of his mother's death, we learn:

God be praised, Coleridge, wonderful as it is to tell, I have never once been otherwise than collected and calm; even on the dreadful day, and in the midst of the terrible scenes I preserved a tranquillity which bystanders may have construed into indifference. . . . I know John will make speeches about it, but she shall not go into a hospital.

Nor did she. Charles undertook the responsibility of caring for his sister and, except for her periodical relapses, when she returned temporarily to the 'mad house', the two lived together until his death, which, contrary to expectations, preceded hers.

The difficult child is, in many cases, exceptionally intelligent, but, owing to some form of maladjustment, is unstable; this instability shows itself in many ways. He is usually an individualist, and finds difficulty in co-operating with his contemporaries; this lack of adjustment may give rise to habits such as bouts of temper, nail-biting, masturbation, exhibitionism and lying, and, in extreme cases, stealing, sadism, masochism and other forms of moral delinquency. These habits are signs of revolt against convention, and may be described as 'mental claustrophobia'. The child is vainly struggling to break through what are often senseless restrictions, and develop some individuality. In these days of small families the child has no opportunity of finding his own level at home. The mother is often over-anxious that the child should be well behaved and does not realize the necessity for making 'mud pies'.

Another type of difficult child is that of the dull or backward. He may develop identical habits as the nervous unstable child but for a different reason. This child is suffering consciously or subconsciously from a sense of inadequacy and blindly tries to compensate for his lack of attainment. It is essential to differentiate between the 'dull' and the 'backward' child, as these two conditions are taken as distinct.[1]

An apparent form of backwardness is the inability to read. This may be due to physical causes, in which case if the cause can be removed the lost ground is quickly recovered. Many children's sight is perfectly normal up to the age of second dentition, when short sight and

[1] 'It should be noted that the phrase is "dull or backward", not "dull and backward", that is, the two conditions are taken as distinct. The terms themselves are not legally or authoritatively defined, but the term "dull" implies a child who is retarded educationally on account of an innate mental inferiority, who will never catch up with his normal fellows and even if placed with a younger class would gradually lose ground. The term "backward" implies one in whom the educational retardation is due to extrinsic causes and who, given special facilities, may catch up or at least be able to keep pace with a group of slightly younger normal children.

'Dullness is commonly due to an all-round subnormality, but may arise from special disabilities such as wandering attention, poor powers of imagery, poor memory, emotional apathy or instability, or to lack of urge or desire for knowledge. There is often rather less inferiority in practical and manual work, so that such children are especially suitable for craft classes.

'Backwardness is more often due to physical handicaps, illness or lowered vitality, or to absence from school, bad conditions in the home, or even to defects in the school organisation; all of which are susceptible of remedy to greater or less extent. It is usual to regard a child who is retarded to the extent of two years in educational attainments as backward.

'For purposes of diagnosis it should be noted that the dull child is retarded all round, his Intelligence Quotient is likely to be from seventy to eighty-five. He exhibits slowness of thought and action, but in subjects which interest him he will show much better results, especially in practical and concrete problems.

'The merely backward child is retarded in educational attainments, but responds well to tests of intelligence, having an Intelligence Quotient of eighty-five or more, and deals with new situations in a common-sense manner.'—*Mental Deficiency Practice*, Shrubsall and Williams.

astigmatism may develop. Parents are sometimes slow to realize that any trouble has arisen in this respect. The child himself may be unaware that his sight is not normal and sees a book as a confused medley of letters, which he hopes in time he will be able to interpret. A child has often a pathetically patient outlook and feels that the inability to overcome any difficulty is due to some fault in himself. This psychological aspect enhances the disability and increases the sense of inadequacy.

It is not always realized by the adult what a tremendous strain is put upon the child who is forced by illness to be absent from school; these absences entail a double amount of work and he is expected to regain the lost ground as well as to keep his place in class. In many cases the teacher makes an attempt to give extra help, but, owing to the size of the classes in most schools, this instruction must perforce be limited.

A child who finds difficulty in reading usually spells badly. Spelling may be learnt and remembered through either the visual or the auditory sense. Many adults on hearing a new word require to see it written rather than hear it spelt.

It often happens that a child may retain a certain amount of baby talk until he begins to learn to read. The visual sense is as a rule as strongly developed as the auditory. The child in 'learning his letters' will in many cases associate the symbol with the correct sound and, if he is taught sympathetically, will with very little mental effort acquire the correct muscular formation, and his speech will quickly become normal for his age. On the other hand, there are many children whose visual memory is undeveloped, and these children may be suffering from a mild form of Alexia. The child should be encouraged to feel the muscular movements of all the sounds and to associate them with the symbol. Where a child has a definite speech defect there is further confusion in the child's mind on being faced with a reading book. He may have been using the substitution 't' for 'k' and has called a cat a 'tat'. In many First Readers a picture is given with the name of the object—the child learns the 'look' of the word and is able to recognize it in a sentence. Now the child has made the same muscular movements for the two consonants, but his visual sense tells him that there are two symbols for the same sound; this will probably cause a confusion which will make him hesitate and a fear arises from it. It is from this moment that great difficulties may arise. This is a very critical stage in the development of the child; if the fear of letters is allowed to go on this may develop into an inhibition regarding his capacity for learning to read. He may develop an intense dislike for reading which will prevent him doing so except under compulsion. A child of this type will never read for pleasure, consequently he will not increase his vocabulary, and at a later stage his ignorance of words may be a very serious handicap. In learning to read a child has to associate symbols with sounds; he has to be able to recognize twenty-six letters which correspond with certain sounds in their simplest form; he has also to understand that these letters represent many other sounds and owing to intricacies of the English spelling he has only his power of visual memory on which to rely. These letters have names, and, in the case of the consonants, a vowel precedes or follows the correct formation of the sound, e.g. 'M' is pronounced 'EM', 'B' is pronounced 'BE'. The vowels cause even greater confusion; the letter 'A' pronounced 'AY' does duty for the sound in mass, pass, and bass (base); in addition the article 'a' can represent two different sounds.

English spelling is complicated owing to various causes. During the reign of King Alfred and for a century and a half after his death Anglo-Saxon was used by the chroniclers in recording historical events and also for dramatic poems. In this respect England was in advance of all other countries, as at this period Latin was universally used for written manuscripts. After the advent of the Normans the language of the country underwent many changes and for a time Norman French and Latin predominated, but by the end of the fourteenth century the English language had re-established itself and the statute of 1362 ordered the use of English instead of French in the pleading of the Law Courts.

The spelling of the language was in no way standardized and was mostly a matter of individual taste, but certain changes of pronunciation in the vowel sounds can be traced back to this period; for instance, the vowel of the word 'hus' was spelt 'ou' by the Normans because of their pronunciation of this vowel 'u', but 'ou' in Anglo-Saxon represented a different sound, consequently the change of the pronunciation of the word 'house'.

The introduction of printing did little to standardize spelling, as the Dutch printers used their imagination drastically in their attempt to reproduce the English sounds. In the seventeenth and eighteenth centuries further complications arose owing to the mistaken philology of the literary men of the day, who, imbued with the classic spirit of that time, imagined that many words of Teutonic and Danish origin were derived from Latin or Greek and altered the spelling to suit their theory.

In the late sixteenth and seventeenth centuries the need for a dictionary made itself felt.

> 'So fine an executant as Dryden, in the last years of his life, announced it as a national scandal that we had yet no English prosody,' nor 'so much as a tolerable dictionary, or a grammar; so that our language is in a manner barbarous'. In 1747 Warburton wrote 'for we have neither Grammar nor Dictionary, neither Chart nor Compass, to guide us through this wide sea of Words'. In 1755 Dr. Johnson published his *English Dictionary and Grammar* and became a great man at once. Merit alone will not explain it; there is a history behind that acclamation. He had made, without help either from Government or from Committees, the book that England had been waiting for and intermittently demanding since the sixteenth century. The long chase, it seemed, was over. Our rebel language was caught up at last; 'Leviathan was hooked.' [1]

Unfortunately Dr. Johnson was influenced by his desire to prove the classical derivation of many homely English words and changed their spelling accordingly. His authority has thus added suffering not only to children but to foreigners endeavouring to learn our language.

It is also often noticeable that the difficult child is gauche and awkward in his movements. The lack of co-ordination which gives rise to language problems is also apparent in lack of rhythm in movement resulting in general clumsiness. This condition is known as apraxia.

> Just as sight and hearing are the two main human senses, so hand-movements and speech—hand-movement guided by the eye and speech appealing to the ear—are the two typical motor activities of mankind. By their means civilized knowledge has been

---

[1] *Shakespeare's English*, George Gordon.

gradually built up, and by their aid it is re-expressed, and re-acquired in each succeeding generation.[1]

Clumsiness, although of physiological origin, is often increased by nervousness; just as to draw attention to a child's speech may increase his difficulties, so unsympathetic criticism of his general movements will increase his awkwardness. Adult criticism should always be constructive, otherwise the sense of inferiority is deepened. The child is innately self-conscious although, in many cases, he tries to hide it by outward manifestation of boisterousness. Defiance and resentment against authority, or a general 'naughtiness', are often symptoms of this same inferiority sense, symptoms in which the victim pretends to glory while inwardly he is miserably aware of failure. In fact they are defence reactions.

A sense of inferiority is inherent, due to the long period of necessary dependence of the child on its parents; the sense of inferiority decreases as the sense of responsibility grows. In some children the feeling of independence develops at a very early age, in others it apparently is lacking. Both these extremes may, through wrong treatment, lead to the creation of the difficult child.

A child who suffers from any form of difficulty of expression, whether visual, oral or auditory, soon realizes his sense of difference from other children, although backwardness in this respect may not be due to any lack of intelligence but may be purely pathological, the psychological aspect of the trouble may have very far-reaching effects, and, in short, may be the *raison d'être* of the difficult child. We are not attempting to cure either the dull or backward by curing his

[1] *The Backward Child*, Cyril Burt.

speech, nor are we suggesting that defective speech will make a child dull or backward, but we do maintain that the renewed hope given by the realization that communication between himself and others can be attained, is of supreme importance in the development of the child's personality.

CHAPTER VIII

The Spoken Word

> A word fitly spoken
> Is like apples of gold in baskets of silver.
>
> PROVERBS

A GENERATION has grown up in our time to which the telephone and the wireless have ceased to be wonders. They are taken for granted. But still less do we pause to wonder at the primary marvel of speech; at words

> Sweet articulate words
> Sweetly divided apart

which in the living voice can take on such intimate and such infinite modulations and which in the masters of speech can become so sensitively alive that they communicate all the subtleties of thought and feeling, from mind to mind and from heart to heart, invisibly but with perfect exactitude. Speech surely is man's greatest achievement. And it is something universal, which concerns us as a necessity from birth to death; I think nothing in education is more fundamental. Especially for us English. We have a glorious language with its wonderful combination of Latin and Saxon, but how few awake to the pleasure that can be got from the fine use of it, from the sound of it even. We muffle and swallow our words, and some people even seem to take a pride in doing it, just as many seem to take a pride in making the signatures to their letters illegible.[1]

Speech does not only consist of words grammatically connected into sentences and pronounced with phonetic

[1] Laurence Binyon's Address to Miss Elsie Fogerty on the presentation of her portrait, 10.x.1937.

correctness, added to these necessary qualities there is something more—the music of the voice. The pleasure given by a beautiful voice is something apart from the enjoyment of the content of the speech; the sound delights our aesthetic sense and we can listen to an unknown language spoken harmoniously with sincere delight. This, however, can only satisfy for a time, soon the need for communication asserts itself, a knowledge of words makes itself manifest and we find that, in addition to inflexion and intonation, we require a knowledge of language and vocabulary.

Inflexion is a subtle quality hard to define, it can convey a hundred different meanings, it can completely change the sense of the words spoken, it can also make clear the environment from which the speaker comes. A foreigner may be phonetically sound perfect in a language, but the slight variations in the intonation of his speech will, at times, betray his origin.

We often read 'In moments of excitement his speech reverted to that of his childhood'; by this we understand that in addition to colloquialisms, the intonation learnt before speech and during its acquirement came back to him. A baby will imitate the type of speech he hears before he can actually repeat words; he listens, desires to produce sounds and learns the lilt of the speech which surrounds him. This power of listening and desire to reproduce new sounds is responsible for that propensity (so much deplored by parents) of the child for picking up the dialect of the county in which he lives.

A child of our acquaintance could sing in perfect tune some months before any words appeared in her speech. We also understand that H.R.H. Princess Margaret sang The Merry Widow waltz at the age of eleven months.[1] In the early days of the First World War a baby, who could not yet speak, was being wheeled in his perambulator on a Common where a squad of soldiers was drilling; the sergeant shouted 'Form Fours', the baby in delight shouted 'AW AW'; the squad collapsed in mirth, the mother in horror. That baby is now a soldier. If there is any connexion between these statements we leave it to others to decide.

To the uninitiated it is a perpetual marvel that soldiers understand and obey the extraordinary sounds emanating from the mouth of the instructor; the advantage of this gift was proved by a subaltern undergoing his promotion examination. The squad was drill perfect and responded nobly to a series of 'Wump-Wumpity—Wumps', the subaltern passed with flying colours but was somewhat nonplussed when his Colonel said, 'Very good, my boy, but you gave one "Wump" too much.'

The inflexion of the voice will convey meaning where words are inaudible, but words are our chief means of communication, so that acquiring of vocabulary, which is the chief aim of the normal child, should also be the ambition of the adolescent and the adult. The normal child of educated parents gradually acquires an extensive vocabulary through imitation and memory; almost unconsciously he learns to speak grammatically and use a clear, well-defined articulation, over a pleasantly modulated voice. The normal child of uneducated parents has often a very hard struggle in his early years; he hears blurred indistinct speech and perforce copies it, with the result that he is often unintelligible to any but his parents until he has been at school for some years. Anyone entering one of the schools in the poorer

[1] *The King's Daughters*, Lady Cynthia Asquith.

8

districts of any of our great towns would be struck by the stupendous task with which the teachers of the Infant classes are faced. Many of the children arrive at school with only the rudiments of speech and have to be taught, not only to acquire new sounds, but to understand a language which appears to them entirely different from that of their parents. In many cases a sense of insecurity arises at this period, due, to no fault of the teacher, but to the child's feeling of bewilderment and inadequacy in the power of communication. This feeling is probably one of the causes of their failure to ask the meaning of words. As these children grow older they often become bilingual, they speak one language in school and another in their homes, they leave school at fourteen and, unless they have the good fortune to associate with children of better understanding, in a few years the school speech is forgotten and the home speech remains.

Children should be encouraged to ask the meaning of words; a healthy intelligent child is often a source of annoyance and embarrassment to his elders by his constant inquiries about the meaning of words; often these inquiries are made at the most inconvenient moments, but a child's world is the present, so the answer is demanded now. 'What is *Holy* Matrimony?' a small boy asked his mother in church! This natural and desirable curiosity seems sadly lacking in many children, whether from indifference, a sense of inadequacy or fear of ridicule it is difficult to say, but it augurs ill for the future development of vocabulary that children of 6 and older can repeat 'Little Miss Muffet' without understanding, either what it was she sat upon or what she was eating. This statement may be doubted, but one of the authors has on several occasions asked classes of children ranging from 6 to 10 what was the meaning of the words 'tuffet' and 'curds and whey'. In the majority of cases tuffet was a mystery; the word was not used in their homes and it appeared to them quite unnecessary to burden themselves with its meaning. The words curds and whey were a complete enigma to all; answers varying from soup to steak and kidney pudding were given. Some of these children were backward though not mentally deficient, but many of them were of normal intelligence. It may be argued that it is only a nursery rhyme and so is unimportant, but it is in these simple rhymes that the foundation of a love of words and their meaning is laid.

Much has been written on the subject of words, their tendency to change in meaning as years go on, in many cases the sense has completely changed. 'Indifferently', 'presently', 'prevent' have altered their meaning since Elizabethan days. In an ancient statute of fines those exempt include 'Lunatics, married women and other incompetent persons'. Certain expressions which are now considered colloquialisms were standard English in former days; if *The Times* announced that 'The Prime Minister blew into the House of Commons', doubtless the Editor would be snowed under by letters from indignant readers, but in 1485 Sir Thomas Malory wrote, 'The knights blew into lodgings', and no one has yet questioned the literary excellence of the *Morte d'Arthur*. In vulgar speech we sometimes 'blot our copy book', but Moses said, 'If not, blot me, I pray thee, out of the book which thou hast written.' When Mistress Page says, 'I cannot tell what the dickens his name is', we feel a glow of pleasure that Shakespeare used slang!

But what is slang? Where is the dividing line between a word of literary value and a colloquialism? New words will always appear in a living language and in every age critics also appear to pour forth vituperation upon these words. The Elizabethans contributed more words than any other age, but some of them suffered much abuse before they were accepted. Sir George Gordon writes:

Court English itself was far from uniform. The noblemen and gentlemen carried their county about with them on their tongues. Sir Walter Raleigh, the pink of elegance, spoke Devon all his life, as Shakespeare, no doubt, spoke Warwickshire. It was even a matter of pride among some of our patriots that this should be so. 'The copiousness of our language', says one of them, 'appeareth in the diversity of our dialects; for we have court, and we have country English, we have Northern and Southern, gross and ordinary, which differ each from other, not only in the terminations, but also in many words, terms, and phrases, and express the same things in divers sorts, yet all write English alike.' This hearty gospel is as far as possible from the old mistaken theory, which modern philology has destroyed, the theory that a language can and should be fixed; that the first duty of a language is to have a polite usage, and that everything else should be for ever impolite; that a civilized language should be commended, like a fashionable club, rather for its power to exclude newcomers than for its willingness to inspect and admit them. The Elizabethans lived before the vogue of this academic theory of language (though one can see it coming), and we, by a similar good fortune, live after its decline. It is a point of community between the Elizabethans and ourselves of which I think we are conscious, and nowhere more warmly than over the language of Shakespeare.[1]

Artificiality or affected speech has always been a source of amusement or ridicule; from time to time arise peculiarities either of pronunciation or expressions which last until they have become stale and then they disappear. One of the earliest criticisms in English on

[1] *Shakespeare's English*, S.P.E. Tract No. XXIX, Sir George Gordon.

such a mannerism is found in the *Canterbury Tales*. Chaucer says of the Frere:

> Somewhat he lisped, for his wantownesse,
> To make his English swete up-on his tonge;

In the middle of the sixteenth century, Pellegrino Morata, the Italian scholar, wrote to his daughter Olympia:

'Pronunciation rather than action is the important point in speaking. The speaker ought to use his lips as the reins of his voice, by which he raises and drops it in turn; he ought to adorn each word before it leaves his palate. But he ought not to do this inelegantly by distorting his lips, puffing out his cheeks, or looking as if he were cracking nuts with his teeth. A lady, before she leaves her chamber, consults her mirror for her expression. The voice ought to do likewise. If it is rough or too sonorous the lips and teeth should be used as barriers to check it; if it is too thin the cheeks should be used to give it animation, if it is too shrill the lips should be drawn together to give it volume, so that the long words be not tripped up by the too delicate palate. Strive that your speech be made pleasant in the speaking. The seductive power of the Goddess of Persuasion, the suavity of Pericles, the bees on the lips of Plato, the chains of Hercules, the lyres of Orpheus and Amphion, the sweetness of Nestor, nay, the grace of Christ himself was nothing else than a sweet, soothing, cheerful, soft speech, not affected nor elaborate, but beautifully delicately, and subtly harmonised. The greatest orator will change the sound not only in every sentence according to its sense, but in every word. I for my part would rather hold my tongue than speak harshly, inarticulately, or unpleasantly.

Throughout his plays, Shakespeare laughs kindly at the rustic speech of his Warwickshire neighbours and ridicules the pedantic utterances of the pedagogue; as Dover Wilson said, 'Shakespeare disliked schoolmasters and they have had their revenge on him ever since.' Fortunately, this revenge is ending and children now read, see, act and consequently love the plays, committing the notes to the place they deserve. Hamlet's advice to the players should be the model for all speech, but that generations of actors playing the name part did not follow it is evident in the north-country expression 'to play 'amlet with 'im'.

We are not told what kind of education was experienced by Mrs. Malaprop, but undoubtedly her understanding of words was not equal to her appreciation of their sound; perhaps her own upbringing displeased her, and caused her to hold such strong views on the proper teaching of young girls.

> But above all, Sir Anthony, she should be mistress of orthodoxy, that she might not mis-spell, and mis-pronounce words so shamefully as girls usually do; and likewise that she might reprehend the true meaning of what she is saying. This, Sir Anthony, is what I would have a woman know—and I don't think there is a superstitious article in it.

Mrs. Malaprop did not appear discomforted by her mistakes, but most people experience a feeling of disquiet after mispronouncing a word; this feeling often restricts the use of words and limits the growth of vocabulary. The love of the meaning of words should be fostered by parents and teachers; unsympathetic treatment of the child's attempt at new words may hamper him through life. He may become completely indifferent to speech except as a necessary method of communication, he may even develop a feeling which might be described as a mental stammer; his speech may be normal, but he mistrusts his knowledge of words and limits himself to an unvaried and familiar vocabulary.

The conversation of many people appears restricted to a few hundred words, and the deficiency in adjectives is made up by the popular expression of the moment; everything from a sweet to Grand Opera is described as 'ripping', 'topping', 'intriguing', 'marvellous', 'wizard' or whatever expletive is 'on duty' at the moment. From time to time a word such as 'gadget' appears, is found to be adequate, and, after trial, is sanctioned by inclusion in the *Oxford Dictionary*. For the most part, however, these expressions sink again into their accustomed place, and the generation which must often have echoed Mistress Quickly's words, 'Here will be abusing of God's patience and the King's English', breathes freely until once more a new term arises to cause fresh discomfort.

This tendency to speak slang has no doubt been deplored by the older generation since speech began, but it must be admitted, however, that undoubtedly a slang word can often convey the meaning vividly if it is used with deliberate intention, instead of, as is usual, with complete disregard of the sense.

The unfortunate result of misusing a slang word can be realized by the following story. A small boy at his first school was having a geography lesson; sitting next to him was a little girl. The question was asked, 'On what river is London?' 'The Thames,' whispered the boy. The little girl put up her hand and said. 'The River Thames.' The next question was 'On what river is Dublin?' 'Gosh!' gasped the boy, so she again put up her hand and said, 'The River Gosh!'

Language is acquired through imitation and word association. A chance word, such as cottage, will conjure up entirely different pictures in the minds of a group of people. This power of visualizing is natural, but it can be encouraged by understanding and tact on the part of parents and teachers. Many words have more than one meaning, a child may get confused

through hearing a word used in another sense; sometimes the result is amusing, sometimes inspired.

After the unexpected death of H.M. King George V,
one of the writers was talking about him to a class of
stammerers; she told them that he was lying in state
in the church at Sandringham, guarded by the men on
the estate. 'But why should he be guarded?' said one
boy, 'no one would want to hurt him.' Surely a fitting
epitaph for the King who, in speech, thought and action
was the guardian of his English.

CHAPTER IX

Progress in Speech Therapy

> When the tongue is paralysed, either from a vice of the organ
> or as a consequence of another disease, and when the patient
> cannot articulate, gargles should be administered of a decoction
> of thyme, hysop, pennyroyal; he should drink water, and the head,
> the neck, mouth, and the part below the chin be well rubbed.
> The tongue should be rubbed with laserwort, and he should chew
> pungent substances, such as mustard, garlic, onions, and make
> every effort to articulate. He must exercise himself to retain his
> breath, wash the head with cold water, eat horse radish, and then
> vomit.
>
> CELSUS: first century A.D.

ALTHOUGH disorders of speech have been noted by
writers in all ages, and have often been a subject for
ridicule, it was not until comparatively lately that the
seriousness of these troubles was recognized by the
Medical and Educational authorities of this country.

During the early nineteenth century certain French
surgeons thought that stammering could be cured by
cutting off portions of the tongue; after several patients
had died, they decided that, although the stammer had
certainly stopped, perhaps this method had obvious dis-
advantages. In the British Museum there are painted
masks used by the 'Devil Dancers' of Ceylon for the
cure of various diseases, including stammering and
deafness.

Sickness is popularly believed to be due to possession by one or more of the various demons of disease, which have to be exorcized to effect a cure. To this end the practitioner (who may have assistants) assumes the costume and masks representing the diseases, and dances the so-called 'devil-dance' (Sanni-yakun-nätima = 'Sickness-demons-dance') in front of the patient with drumming and invocations. The dancing may be continued, if necessary, throughout the night; the demon is then believed to have left the sufferer and entered into the body of the masked dancer, who thereupon rushes, or is driven from the scene. Each of the demons of disease has its appropriate mask, distinguished both by its colours and features. In some of them the characterization is more obvious than in others, e.g. red for 'fever', yellow for 'biliousness', eyes without pupils for 'blindness', or a distorted mouth for stammering.[1]

Many methods have been tried in the cure of stammering, we are all familiar with the story of Demosthenes and the pebble. We know that Moses was a stammerer, and that he refused, at first, to lead the Jewish revolt against the Egyptians on account of his stammer. It seems almost certain that when he had once assumed the leadership, that his sense of inadequacy ceased, and he lost his fear of speech.

That stammering was a serious disorder which required treatment was recognized during the later years of the last century, especially on the Continent, but very little was done in this country until a few years before the 1914–18 war. The many speech disorders, which are now recognized under separate categories, were not formerly considered to be due to different causes.

In 1912 the first Conference in Speech Training was held in London. Dr. Crichton Miller read a paper on stammering which first formulated the theory in England of the psychological causation of stammering. Miss Elsie Fogerty, in conjunction with the authorities

[1] British Museum Publications, set B.49.

of one of the largest London hospitals, was responsible for the opening of one of the first clinics for speech disorders. Several other hospitals started speech work about this time.

During the 1914–18 war more and more people recognized the fact that stammering was a nervous disorder and not a speech defect. Many men with a neuropathic history suffering from shell-shock developed a stammer, and its incidence was increased among children living in air-raid districts. In 1917 an experimental clinic for stammerers was opened in Westminster by Miss Elsie Fogerty. The object was to bring to the notice of the Educational Authorities the prevalence of this distressing affliction among our children and the fact that definite and scientific means were available to combat it. The experiment was completely successful and, in 1918, the London County Council opened its first four Centres for Stammerers. During the next few years the number was increased.

While the centres in London were increasing, clinics were being formed for speech disorders by other County and Borough Authorities, and at least one clinic was opened before the London Centres were formed. In 1931 the Central Association of Mental Welfare appointed a Travelling Speech Therapist. In addition to the speech work among the mentally defective, she undertook to diagnose and advise upon children suffering from various forms of defective speech in schools under the local Education Authorities. As a result of this work more and more Authorities in the Provinces appointed a whole- or part-time Speech Therapist.

In June, 1933, the Stockton Education Committee submitted the following resolution to the Association of Education Committees' Conference at Brighton:

That in view of the serious handicap to children with defective speech (stammering, etc.), and of the success that has attended the efforts made by certain education authorities to remove such disabilities, the Executive Committee of the Association of Education Committees be urged to press upon the Government the desirability of making provision for meeting the special needs of such children compulsory.

In 1934 the Mental Hospital Committee appointed a Speech Therapist at two of their principal Certified Institutions. Attention was drawn to the fact that the inability of the Mental Defective to communicate with his fellows is a source of inadequacy and inferiority; it was felt that if he could be taught to speak at least fairly well it would give him a sense of well-being that would help him to attempt to make a success of a life that had hitherto been a failure. At the same time a Speech Therapist was appointed to a London County Council Residential Home for Mentally Defective Children. Some time after this another Certified Institution appointed a Speech Therapist.

In 1935 classes were started for speech disorders at a London County Council Training Colony for the Unemployed. Some years ago speech clinics were opened in Edinburgh, Glasgow and Ulster; since then the work has increased greatly and centres have been opened in other large towns.

The constant flow of visitors from overseas emphasizes the fact, if any emphasis is necessary, of the widespread interest and need for this work.

Until recently treatment by relaxation was confined to stammerers, but proof has now been made of the value of muscular relaxation preceding, and coinciding with, the speech training required in the specific defect. A child of 9 suffering from a lisp was intensely sensitive about her defect, her nervous condition was such that for several months her only treatment was relaxation. At the end of that time the lisp had practically disappeared and her speech required only a little adjustment to become normal.

During the last few years very interesting experiments have been made at two of the Certified Institutions for Mentally Defectives among the Epileptic patients. In all organic defects there is a varying amount of superimposed tension; if this can be relieved by relaxation the condition of the patient improves. Although relaxation may diminish the frequency and severity of the fits, it is not claimed to be a definite cure, but anything that will alleviate this distressing condition is worth while. A marked improvement in the expression and demeanour of the patients after relaxation is apparent, and in many cases a reduction of fits has been noticed in the official charts. The circulation of one patient was so bad that her arms and fingers were often 'dead' when she came for treatment. Gradually the circulation improved, the fits became less frequent, and at the end of two years she was allowed to return home and go out to domestic service.

The majority of the patients in the Mental Hospitals show appreciation and a desire to co-operate. One exception was a boy of 18, a stammerer, who, after attending three times, told the Medical Superintendent that the speech work was a 'wash out' and that he could cure himself. He was allowed to absent himself, but six months later he returned to the class of his own accord and eventually his stammer was cured. He was allowed out on licence and is now doing well.

Another case may be of interest; a girl of 18 with paralysis of the whole of the right side of the body had an acute stammer accompanied by severe facial spasm. Her attempts to speak were most painful, and she had a most unhappy expression. Under treatment the pained look left her face, the spasm disappeared, the stammer became less and she began to smile. Six months later she was able to use the fingers of her right hand; the super-imposed tension had been relieved by relaxation, although the organic defect was incurable.

It has been noticed that with improved speech increased stability has been obtained, resulting in improved behaviour and more equable temper.

The work at the Training Centre for the Unemployed is another instance where speech training is of social service. The majority of these men are suffering from a twofold sense of inadequacy due to their imperfect speech and long-standing lack of employment. Many come from outlying districts where they had no opportunity of obtaining treatment during their schooldays. In addition to the actual speech trouble, there is, in many cases, a self-consciousness regarding their lack of vocabulary, which intensifies the fear of speech. Many of them almost despair of ever getting any permanent work. One man, aged 30, a lisper, suffering from congenital facial paralysis, had been in institutions all his life and had lost hope of ever getting work, although he was anxious to do so. Owing to his paralysis, the visiting Medical Officer did not consider it likely that much could be done for his speech defect, but in a month he was able to whistle; his speech and self-confidence improved so much that he obtained work as a houseman at one of the great Public Schools.

A great number of these men have lost touch with their relations, and consequently have lost their sense of social obligation; the physical and mental relief which results from relaxation, and the sympathetic interest in their personal concerns, are important factors in their psychological readjustment. The men enjoy discussing the social activities, of which there are many, in the colony. A large proportion of these men have obtained work, three of them being accepted in H.M. Forces.

It seems incredible that a man should lose his job because he stammers, but unfortunately it is still only too true. Some time ago a Medical Officer was visiting a Casual Ward and asked the Welfare Officer if he had met many stammerers in the course of his duties. He was told that among some thousands of casuals very few had been noticed. As things turned out, the next case the Medical Officer saw was a very severe stammerer; he asked the man whether his speech was really a drawback to his getting work. The man denied it strenuously as he did not know that his questioner was a doctor, but thought that he ought to make a good impression on a prospective employer. They had a long talk and eventually the man admitted that he had lost his job on account of his stammer. The man was inspired with hope and the thought of something in the way of work seemed to give him confidence, so much so that even after such a short time he spoke with less stammer. Arrangements were made to get him employment and treatment for his speech.

In 1934 the Association of Teachers of Speech and Drama formed a Section for Remedial Speech, later known as the Association of Speech Therapists. In 1935 the British Society of Speech Therapists was formed. Both these societies were recognized by the Board of Registration of Medical Auxiliaries. In 1945 the amalgamation of the two societies was completed and the College of Speech Therapists came into being, and in 1948 H.M. the King graciously conferred Royal Patronage.

The College is the official examining body for entry into the profession. At present there are four training schools in England and two in Scotland, but it is hoped that more will be formed in the near future.

Conferences and courses have been held from time to time, and in 1948 the College was host to the International Conference of Speech Therapists; it was the first meeting of this body since the war and delegates came from all over the world.

During the Second World War much work was undertaken by speech therapists in hospitals all over the British Isles for the rehabilitation of men suffering from war injuries. In 1947 the first residential school for small children suffering from certain speech disorders was opened at Moor House, Surrey.

If at any time we thought that speech was an isolated factor in development, that idea has long ceased to exist. The deeper we get in this work the more we realize that speech affects and is affected by everything in the personality. A nervous disorder will have a deleterious effect on speech, and a speech disorder an equally disturbing influence on the nervous system. Some time ago a Speech Clinic was opened at a Hospital for Children in London, and shortly after it was opened it was found necessary to divide the work into two departments, one for children suffering from functional and organic speech disorders, and the other for children suffering from enuresis, nail-biting, sleep-walking, bad temper and other nervous habits.

Although a great deal has been done in this country during the last quarter of a century, speech therapy is still in the experimental stage, and research must go on in every branch of this subject. We should like to feel that the fable of La Fontaine, in which an agriculturist consulted a sage, is applicable to the work of the Speech Therapist. The sage commanded him to search diligently over his field to a depth of two feet and there he would find an amulet; when he had found it his crops would flourish apace. He did not find the amulet, but as a result of his unusual digging—for he was a lazy man—he had a bumper harvest. Similarly, we hope in our efforts at treatment that we are doing more than removing the child's speech disorder; we are attempting to alter his mental outlook, release him from his purgatory and open up vistas of a new world.

MILESTONES

1906. Classes for stammering children in Manchester.

1911. Speech Clinic at St. Bartholomew's Hospital.

1913. Speech Clinic at St. Thomas' Hospital.

1914. L.C.C. Evening Institutes for Stammerers.

1918. First L.C.C. County Council School Speech Clinic. Appointment of salaried speech therapist by War Office.

1923. Research undertaken at University College.

1924. Research undertaken at King's College Hospital.

1931. Travelling Speech Therapists appointed by Central Association for Mental Welfare.

1932. Students admitted to L.C.C. Speech Centres.

1934. Speech Therapists appointed to Hospitals for Mental Defectives.

1942. Registration of Speech Therapists with B.R.M.A.

1945. First Meeting of College of Speech Therapists. Speech Therapy for school children suffering from speech disabilities made a statutory obligation under Education Act of 1944.

1947. College Examinations held for first time. Opening of Moor House School.

1948. His Majesty the King graciously confers Royal Patronage on College.

Statistics

IT has been suggested that treatment of speech defects among the mentally defective was not worth while, but it has been found that apart from the actual treatment of the defect in question there is no doubt that this therapy has a marked socializing effect on the patient.

Some years ago an experiment was carried out on high-grade defectives who were stammerers; eight cases were treated. As a result of this experiment three cases improved sufficiently to be sent out on licence. Shortly afterwards the authorities decided to explore the possibilities of a more intensive campaign, and investigations were carried out at two large Certified Institutions for the Mentally Defective with the following results:

				Male.	Female.	Improv-able.	Not Improv-able.
1.	Children	.	. 350	147	46	193	157
	Adults .	.	. 90	22	18	40	50
2.	Children	.	. 18	8	2	10	8
	Adults .	.	. 85	16	24	40	45

The children have been classified in the following categories:

Institution I.

Class.	No.	Stammering.	Lisping.	Lalling.	Cleft Palate.	Phonaesthenia.	Velum defects.	Rhinolalia.	Echolalia.	Improvable.	Not Improvable.
I.	23	1	1	8	1					11	1
IA.	23	1	3		1	2	2			14	
IIA.	22	2	4			2	2			12	
II.	26	1	11	3		1				10	
IIIA.	22		8					3		11	
IIIB.	24	1	12			1		1	1	8	
III.	25		5	3		1		3		12	
IVA.	22	2	8	1				1		6	4
IV.	25	2	8		1		1	1		8	4
VA.	26	2	6	7		2		2		7	
V.	24		5	7		1	2	9			
VIA.	23	1	8	5		2	1			6	
VI.	24	2	6	5						11	
VII.	19	2	4	4					1	1	7
VIIA.	22	Imbeciles, difficult to grade.									22

Institution II.

	10		3	5						2	

Some of the nurses in these institutions were particularly interested in this work and volunteered to carry out the exercises given by the therapist, between visits. As a result the speech-therapy work was markedly enhanced.

Shortly after the investigation of the speech of the Mentally Defective in Certified Institutions was carried out, the same type of examination was made in two of the Special Schools. The children in these schools are on average of a higher grade, and it is interesting to note the comparison between their speech and that of those in the Certified Institutions. The figures are small but they give some indication of the speech in Special Schools.

1. SPECIAL SCHOOL FOR BOYS

No.	St.	Lisp.	Lall.	C.P.	Velum Defects.	Rhin.	Imp. M.D. Speech.	Normal Speech
100	2	14	10		9	20	40	5

2. SPECIAL SCHOOL FOR GIRLS

No.	St.	Lisp.	Lall.	C.P.	Velum Defects.	Rhin.	Imp. M.D. Speech.	Normal Speech
100	1	10	12	1	6	5	60	5

In all the cases examined there were a large proportion of children who had no special defect but whose intonation was dull and lifeless, which is a very common occurrence where the mind is impaired. Many of these cases are capable of improvement under tuition; this fact has been proved by the work that has since been carried out in a Special School.

We should like to refer to the great interest that has been taken in America in Speech Therapy. In California, we understand that every school of a certain size has a speech therapist on its staff. We quote from a very interesting article by Miss Emily Clegg Halls, writing in *The Indiana Teacher*, April, 1936.

A recent survey of Indiana school children handicapped in speech, under the direction and co-operation of Indiana University Psychological Department at Riley Hospital and State Superintendent of Public Instruction, revealed the fact that at least twenty-three thousand children in the grades from 1B through high school come under one of the three following classes of speech disorders—stutterers, cleft palates or infantile cases. If this condition was revealed in a general survey, what would it show if it were possible to have a personal, scientific examination of every child in our public school, by educators trained in this special field?

We quote from the Preliminary Report on the Indiana Speech Survey by Dr. C. M. Louttit, director of Clinical Psychology at Indiana University.

A report on speech defects included in a volume, *Special Education; the Handicapped and the Gifted*, published as one of the volumes from the White House Conference on Child Health and Protection, and prepared by Drs. Robert West, Lee E. Travis and Miss Pauline B. Camp, was based on a questionnaire survey in cities of over 10,000 population. This report was sent to all cities of over 10,000 population, but contained no data received from any community in Indiana. Perhaps we do not have any speech defects. It is our problem to find out.

The task of securing data on the number of speech defective children throughout the whole state is a difficult one. Perhaps the ideal would be an individual examination of every child, but is obviously impossible. As the only practicable way, we decided to request data from each principal, who in turn would secure the figures from each classroom teacher. Therefore, our data are based on the teacher's observation. A one-sheet blank was prepared, and after revision was sent to county or city superintendents through the office of the State Superintendent of Public Instruction.

As far as we are aware, blanks were furnished to the principals of each of 3,717 public schools of the state. One thousand two hundred and twenty-three of these blanks were returned from schools with a total pupil population of 315,353. As was to be expected, not all of these blanks are in usable form. Reports for two-thirds of the total population were completed. From most of the other one-third the data was not distributed by sex or grade, and about one per cent had to be eliminated entirely. We have no means of demonstrating the reliability of our data. Teacher's judgement is the basis of the raw figures. Where schools were obviously in error, as one school with 16 pupils reported 16 stutterers or another of 64 pupils with 35 cleft palates, they were eliminated. In a population of some 200,000 it is probable chance errors in teacher's observation have been ironed out.

The school systems of the state were about one-half covered by the reports received. Fifty-four of 92 county and 51 of 104 city systems returned blanks for all or part of their schools. Total number of children covered in complete reports 199,839, or about 27 per cent of the school children of the state.

The reports, on cursory examination, represent a fair geographical distribution. It would thus appear that our sample is sufficiently large to be representative. The incomplete blanks represent another 15 per cent, but their data could not be used in our subsequent analyses, because they lack certain data.

Calculations based upon complete reports alone show the city system to have 3·3 per cent, county system 4·3 per cent, with a total incidence of 3·7 per cent.

Sex differences are decidedly in evidence. In both city and

county schools the percentage of boys with defects is one and one-half times as great as the percentage of girls. For the total group there were 4·6 per cent of the boys and 2·7 per cent of the girls. Race differences were not so evident. Basing figures on schools reporting wholly Negro, we find 3·8 per cent with defects compared with 3·3 per cent for total group. The incidence of speech defects in special classes for the mentally subnormal is high. Twenty-three schools reported one or more special subnormal classes with a total of 855 children, 520 boys and 335 girls. Of the boys 9·9 per cent and of girls 11·3 per cent exhibited speech defects, giving a total incidence of 10·6 per cent.

For the moment we shall disregard the total population and consider only children with speech defects. In the new first graders, 84 per cent show articulatory disorders and only 9 per cent are stutterers; while in the twelfth grade, 31·5 per cent still show articulatory troubles, and 56 per cent are stutterers.

While we recognized the limitations of our data, still we are able to get a clearer idea of the extent of the problem of speech defective children in our public schools of this state. Special attention to children's speech in the first grade would correct most of the problems before they can interfere with child's adjustment.

Data of Child Development

(Taken from Publication No. 91, Children Bureau, U.S. Department of Labour)

WE have discussed the problem of arrested development and the various disorders which may arise therefrom both in the normal and the sub-normal child. We should like to include in this appendix the summary of the attainments of the intelligent child.

1. INFANCY—first twelve months of life

   (a) MOTOR DEVELOPMENT—

     Eyes—

       By 3 weeks eyes are fixed on bright stationary objects.

       At 4 weeks they travel from one object to another.

       At 5 weeks they follow slightly moving objects.

       At 8 weeks they are accommodated to distance.

       Eye movements should be complete within the first 12 weeks.

     Head and Trunk—

       At 4 weeks the child will take the nipple with his lips.

       At 8 weeks the head is held up but is very wobbly at first.

       By 9 weeks the back is straightened.

       By 12 weeks an effort is made to sit up.

       By 24 weeks he sits up alone.

By 6 months he learns to bite his toes, at 8 months
he can get on his hands and knees, and by
9 months he begins to creep.

Hands—

At 9 weeks the child joins his hands together.

By 10 weeks hands are put to the mouth.

By 2 months the child begins to explore objects
which the hands chance to touch without looking at the object.

By 19 weeks, grasping is developed.

By the 22nd week objects are held in the hand and
looked at before going into the mouth.

By 26 weeks objects are picked up accurately.

At 6 months imitative movements are begun.

At 9–10 months hands are very active.

At 11 months right-handedness becomes evident.

At 12 months imitation is well developed.

Feet and legs—

At 8–9 weeks the child begins to push hard with
his legs.

From 12 weeks on this develops and efforts are
made by the child to be supported with his feet
touching the lap.

From 14 weeks on the movements are rhythmic
in response to music, this is often described as
'dancing'.

At 6 months he will push forward with his feet and
move on hands and knees.

At 8 months he will lie on his back with legs free
and throw legs upwards and bring them down
hard, the movement being often repeated.

About 9 months he pulls himself up to a standing
position and can stand steadied by one hand.

By $9\frac{1}{2}$ months he can stand alone for a short period
without support.

By 10 months he can edge along by a chair.

By 11 months he can walk by pushing a baby-car or chair.

At 12 months he commences to walk alone.

(b) SENSORY DEVELOPMENT—

Vision—

At 12 weeks there is a recognition of faces.

At 13 weeks the child looks for an object which has disappeared.

At 19 weeks an object is reached for when noticed.

Between 16 and 24 weeks there is obvious great enjoyment in merely looking around.

Hearing and Voice—

Almost from the start there is recognition of loud sounds.

At 4 weeks attention is paid to sounds such as those of a piano.

At 7–8 weeks the child smiles in response to voices.

At about 13 weeks he turns to look in the direction of sounds.

At about 17 weeks experiments are made in producing sounds.

At about 21 weeks the child laughs at such sounds as a snapping towel.

By 7 months the names of the members of the family seem to be recognized.

By 9 months the meaning of 'no—no' is known.

Between 9 and 10 months a few words appear to possess meaning.

At 10 months sounds with meanings are made, one to call attention, one of negation and one of desire.

During the second 6 months considerable powers of attention are displayed and may last for many minutes. At about 6 months the child takes an interest in watching things fall, recognizes the sight of his perambulator and of his mother with her hat on and interprets these to mean that he is going out, and looks up when the names of members of the family are spoken.

Emotion—

The child begins to show fear from a very early period.

From 1 to 6 weeks there is convulsive recognition of loud sounds, and will struggle and cry if held so that free movement is impeded.

By 6 weeks the child smiles and shows signs of contentment.

Between 7 and 8 weeks he will smile in response to voices.

From 8 to 12 weeks he shows signs of satisfaction in looking at new objects.

From 12 to 16 weeks he laughs loud when played with.

At 21 weeks he laughs loud at explosive sounds.

At 12–16 weeks the child shows signs of fear on seeing strangers, and will cry and grow stiff if compelled to lie down when he wishes to try to sit up.

At $7\frac{1}{2}$ months he shows signs of joy at the sight of his perambulator or hat.

At $8\frac{1}{2}$ months there is unwillingness to being picked up by strangers, he cries to go to his mother, and cries if he has not her undivided attention.

By 9 months he cries if laughed at.

2. THE PRE-SCHOOL CHILD—1–5 Years

(*a*) MOTOR ACTIVITIES—

At 18 months the process of walking is perfected.

Soon after the child learns to sit on a chair and rhythmic motion in response to music becomes well developed.

At 16 months the child can put a spoon into its mouth.

By 18 months he can eat with a spoon without much spilling and can hold a glass with both hands and drink from it.

At 5 years or a little later a knife and fork can be used.

At 15 months the child can play 'go shopping'.

At about 17½ months he begins to cut with scissors.

At 18 months he imitates domestic scenes, pouring out tea and coffee, wipes the floor, washes doll's face and hands.

Between 1½ and 2 years he is able to open and shut lids of boxes and drawers.

At 2 years he can build with blocks.

At 2½ years he impersonates an animal or another person.

Between 3 and 5 years play largely takes the form of make-believe. He plays all the adult activities he has the chance to observe. He loves to repeat the same game in the same way again and again. At this period play tends to become solitary or with adults. There is little ability to play with children of the same age.

At 4 years the child uses scissors effectively, and he can follow an outline roughly with a pencil.

At 5 years people and objects are drawn crudely.

At 18 months the child has become clean.

By 2 years the child has become dry though control of the bladder at night may not be acquired till 3 years.

By 3–4 years the child can dress and undress simply and begins to manipulate hooks and buttons.

At 4–5 years he had learned to brush his teeth.

(*b*) SENSORY ACTIVITIES—

At 15 months the child compares objects and may recognize photographs.

At 18 months he can find pictures in a book on hearing its name or the rhyme which refers to it.

At 20 months he can point out hair, eyes, &c., in pictures.

Between 2 and 3 years delight is taken in looking at pictures.

The child understands words before he begins to speak. The order of acquisition of words depends on interests and activities. He learns rapidly words which are cues to action. He first learns the names of persons, then objects, and finally qualifying words (big, hot, &c.). Colour names are learned late. Children of a silent mother or brought up in institutions learn slowly.

At 18 months the most common words of everyday life should be understood; a single word often conveys the meaning of a sentence.

At 18 months–2 years phrases and very simple sentences are used.

At 3 years sentences in complete form are used and rhymes are memorized.

At 4 years a child can fit a round block in a round hole and a square block in a square hole, &c., without trial.

Up to 4 years concepts of time are very vague, yesterday and to-morrow—breakfast, dinner and supper—may be confused.

Between 4 and 6 years a child acquires correct concepts of past and future and of morning and afternoon, but remains vague as to weeks, months and years.

At from 5 to 6 years the average child begins to realize that printed words may stand for real objects and may attempt to read. At this age he wants to read the same story over and over again.

(c) REASONING—

At 4 years logical processes of thought have quite definitely commenced and ability to distinguish between dreams and realities develops.

Between 5 and 6 years a child can distinguish between an imagined event and a real past event. The first permanent consecutive memories that can be spontaneously recalled in later life usually date back to this period (4–6 years).

(d) EMOTIONAL DEVELOPMENT—

At 1–2 years tantrums are likely to occur.

At 18 months a child shows sympathy for a chair which has been knocked over, and feeds the doll. Jealousy, sensitiveness to ridicule, resentment and a desire to please develop during these years.

From 3 to 6 years the child becomes definitely conscious of his personality and sets himself off against the world, deliberately trying to see how far he can safely defy adults. The child is particularly susceptible to suggestions at this age.

In the earlier years a child responds more readily to negative than to positive suggestion (e.g. a child of 4 years refused to eat rice when urged, but afterwards cried for it when told he could not have it).

At this age a child shows an enjoyment of secrets.

This is due to a dawning realization that the content of his consciousness is not immediately accessible to other people.

The Relation between Defective Speech and Disability in Spelling

(*Fred J. Schonell in 'The British Journal of Educational Psychology'*)

DURING the course of investigations on the disability of spelling among London elementary school children F. J. Schonell writes that

there arose two allied, but not so fundamentally important, problems, firstly, 'How far is there a relation between inaccurate spelling and mispronunciation?' and secondly, 'What influence has stammering on spelling ability?' Little information existed on these problems, hence towards the close of the major investigation they were considered in some detail. The combined results obtained from the various sources provide clear and comprehensive knowledge of an experimental nature on the entire question of defective speech and disability in spelling. Throughout the investigation there was ample evidence that faulty pronunciation was a prolific contributory cause of mis-spelling. Naturally, it was never the major or sole causal factor in a case of backwardness, but it was observed that if a child constantly pronounced inaccurately he not infrequently spelt inaccurately, and the nature of his written errors bore remarkable similarity to the nature of his spoken errors.

Thirdly, the spelling error due essentially to mispronunciation is more prevalent amongst boys than girls—the proportion in the cases studied was 21·8 per cent to 10 per cent. No doubt this is a further manifestation of that characteristic of tidiness and attention to detail which one finds more strongly developed in girls than boys. The girls, more attentive to tidy habits in dress and work, is also more concerned with tidiness in speech.

Fourthly, those who rely on auditory recall are apt to be led astray by faulty pronunciation more frequently than those whose recall is by a visual means.

SUMMARY OF CONCLUSIONS

1. In an investigation on speech defects and spelling ability it was found that organic defects were much less frequent than functional ones. A speech defect which is at first organic can, even after the cause of the defect has been removed, leave behind it a set of faulty speech habits which have a detrimental influence on attainments in spelling and reading.

2. Speech defects are a cause of backwardness in spelling and reading on account of the handicap they occasion in setting up a foundation of accurate articulatory-auditory units, a mode of learning and recall which is very much used by young children. Such a handicap is greatly accentuated for those children when too much emphasis is placed on phonic methods and insufficient on visual and kinæsthetic.

The causes of a child's faulty pronunciation were three:

(a) Bad environmental influences of home and companions.

(b) Habitual lip laziness.

(c) Shyness and inferiority attitude resulting in mumbling, slurring, and clipping words when reading and speaking.

The factors affecting the incidence of mistakes in spelling due to mispronunciation were fourfold. Firstly, this type of error was commonest amongst children from schools of poor social grade. Secondly, younger children were more prone to them than older children. Young children actually say the words aloud when they write,[1] so that there is greater likelihood of pronunciation errors becoming spelling errors. As familiarity with words increases and the mechanics of writing become almost automatic there is less reliance on the articulatory motor and auditory aids and more on the visual and grapho-motor aids. From actually saying the words he passes to an abbreviated form of articulation and thence to 'inner speech', when no movement of the lips is perceptible or

---

[1] The same characteristic is observed during silent reading, but whereas vocalization is in many cases a hindrance to speed and occasionally to efficiency of comprehension, accurate vocalization during spelling, especially of long and unfamiliar words, is definitely an aid.

sound audible, but where there is in most cases a slight movement of the tongue, the soft palate or some other portion of the vocal organs. Some of the shortcomings in accurate speech of seven, eight and nine-year-olds disappear with age; a child might write ferver (further) and eneyfink (anything) at eight, but not at ten.

3. Intense functional paraphemia was the speech defect which was the most potent cause of disability in spelling; it was the major causal factor in the meagre verbal achievements of four out of 105 cases of specific backwardness. This defect which is due to a lowered power of auditory discrimination in the realm of speech, manifests itself in the pupil's inability to differentiate between phonic elements of similar value, such as 'ch' and 'sh', 'k' and 'ch', 'f' and 'v'. Although the cases studied could hear and understand spoken words perfectly, had a good vocabulary, and could converse intelligently provided one became familiar with their inarticulate speech, yet their attainments in spelling and reading were below mental age expectations to the extent of 2 years in the least pronounced and 4½ years in the most pronounced case.

4. In every case of speech defect there was evidence of accompanying emotional inhibitions and consequent loss of confidence, which to some extent affected ability in reading, spelling, and composition.

5. Stammering appears to hinder normal achievements in spelling only in children where the extent and severity of their nervous instability are serious. That is, stammering exerts its influence in a general and not a specific manner; it is never a cause of specific disability in spelling. There are almost as many cases upon whom the defect has no influence as there are those for whom it is a possible cause of inaccurate spelling.

6. The misspelling of some stammerers shows one characteristic error, namely, the tendency to lengthen the word by the addition of a superfluous consonant.

7. Faulty pronunciation is a minor contributory force in the spelling backwardness of some children.

Notes on Some Cases of Word Blindness

(Elsie Fogerty, C.B.E., L.R.A.M., Superintendent, Speech Clinic, St. Thomas's Hospital, London, England)

WORD Blindness or Alexia has been attributed by Ferrier, Monk and Wyllie to a disorder of the visual word 'Centre', including the Angular Convolution and the Supra-Marginal Convolution. Two classes of the defect have been distinguished:

(1) those in which the patient is at the same time agraphic;

(2) those in which the patient though word-blind is not agraphic; one being due to destruction, and the other only to subordinate lesion, of the connexion between the primary visual centres and the higher visual word centre. It is obviously outside my proper sphere to discuss any of these conclusions; but I would venture to suggest that they were in the main the result of investigation in adult cases of a pathological character. Such seems to have been the case in the classical work of Dejerine and Serieux quoted by Dr. Wyllie in his *Disorders of Speech*.[1]

The close investigation of word blindness in young children during recent years and the modification in the general theory of the relation of speech to certain brain centres admits a doubt whether some other types of Alexia may not exist in which a more purely functional disturbance

---

[1] Pp. 333–49.

can be distinguished; it is in relation to certain cases of the kind that the following paper is presented. No attempt has been made to theorize on any anatomical or physiological conditions involved, and where the term 'centre' is used it is employed merely to indicate a definite and perceptible point in the normal course of the afferent and efferent paths in a speech impulse.

It is obvious that in Alexia the failure takes place between the visual centre in 'looking' at the written word and the specific speech centres, sensory and motor.

Two types of cases have been kept under observation and treated for fairly continuous periods:

(A) Cases in young children sometimes exhibiting symptoms of general mental deficiency. In no case given here has the character of this deficiency been grave enough to place the child definitely on the certifiable list.

(B) One case which was afterwards definitely certified and which was accompanied by complete asphasia.

(C) Cases of children and young adults showing a high type of intelligence in whom more or less complete Alexia existed. In the older cases very complete investigations have been made of the patients' visual condition and in each case it has been decided that no form of mechanical help by glasses promised any relief.

The following five cases illustrate the observations made and the methods employed in overcoming the defect.

I (J. R.)—8 years of age, sent to the Speech Clinic of a London hospital as mentally deficient; slight stammer; quite unable to read; clever with his hands; very backward at school. General observation showed a keen intelligent sense of humour, great capacity for remembering commands and even complicated directions; completely reasonable action in all his ordinary proceedings; as the treatment continued he became the monitor of the class and showed quick intelligence in all his duties. At this time (1913) word blindness was generally regarded as giving little promise of results from treatment. J. R.'s inability to distinguish letters was profound. He had picked up some of the names in his school experience, but cheerfully presented Z, W and D as hopeful candidates for the letter A.

Before leaving the Clinic he could write quite fairly well, read his own writing without difficulty—this is frequently found in cases in Alexia—he read the names of all objects he was sent to fetch, and even at times was found reading to himself. His case was one of those of which track was lost during the War.

II (E. L.)—8 to 12. This case was charmingly friendly and intelligent, conversed quite sensibly and was able to earn money as a small errand-boy, but was found hopeless at school. He read not at all and wrote with a good deal of difficulty, spoke well and drew very much better than most boys of his age. Methods of treatment had developed considerably by this time and E. L. soon learned to recognize all letters, spell words with block letters, read ordinary words, print block letters and write fairly well. He had no love of reading, differing in this from J. R., but he could read ordinary sentences quite intelligently and distinguish addresses, shop signs, &c. He was successful in his work as an errand-boy, but did not show great intelligence at any time. He still attends at intervals for revision of his work and maintains progress.

III (A. B.)—One of the older girls at a well-known Girls' public school. A clever artist, taking up drawing as a profession, completely word-blind. Wrote fairly well and could generally read what she had written, great care having been expended on her education. She had private lessons and before leaving read practically normally. When last seen she reported that she was hardly troubled at all by her defect.

IV (O. L.)—A somewhat similar case, hampered all her

life by word blindness. She came of a very brilliant family and had been carefully educated by being read to. Her writing was fair but she found difficulty in reading it. Her word blindness was practically complete in reading print. She had received particularly accurate optical attention and the case had been pronounced to be purely one of word blindness. She was a most energetic and careful student and followed her exercises conscientiously. There were ultimately no remaining signs of any real difficulty in reading, though her sentence stressing was rather uncertain and slow. She has continued her practice and may be counted as a cure.

V (M. G.)—A young girl of Italian race particularly gifted as a speaker. She is now among the most successful students of a leading dramatic school. She has an excellent verbal memory, and is a remarkably fine verse speaker. When first seen at about 14 years of age she could with difficulty distinguish letters but was quite unable to read words. After over two years' treatment she was able to take her place in ordinary rehearsal classes, reading her parts and learning them very easily from the script. When nervous her reading aloud is still poor and she is unsuccessful in this part of her diction tests. She writes quite well and reads to herself without difficulty.

Among the difficulties which have been met with in the treatment of children attending primary schools the greatest is the fact that they have lost step with their contemporaries in learning to read. The child whose word blindness has been completely overcome is still in a measure in the same position as the normal child who has just learned to read. The reading vocabulary is small, sentence stress is uncertain, and there is no natural love of reading to induce constant voluntary practice. When these children return to the normal school class, where their contemporaries in age now have no further teaching in reading, they are often reported 'to read no better than they did before'. What is needed here is a special practice class for such cases, as it is difficult to keep them long enough at the clinic to ensure complete fluency, and their own school teachers are better trained in the devices for teaching reading than the majority of clinicians.

1. The first exercise given is Blind Reading. Very solid wooden block letters are employed, the child standing with his back to the teacher, a letter is placed in his hand held behind the back. The name of the letter is then given and the peculiarities of the shape described. This is continued without any use of sight until all the letters can be named phonically and alphabetically: 'its name is Pee, and it says Puh, &c.'

2. The process is repeated while the child draws a rough sign for the letter in the air with the forefinger.

3. The process is repeated but after naming each letter the child looks at it and puts it down in front of him.

4. The child is now asked not to name the letter until *after* he has looked at it, and where this is not successfully done he returns to the blindfold feeling.

5. The child looks at the letter, names it and tests the correctness of his impression by feeling the letter.

6. Block letter drawing is now introduced, and all the impressions are compared and used in haphazard order, e.g. look at it, draw it, name it, feel it, sound it.—Look at it, sound it, draw it, name it, feel it, &c., &c.

7. Very large printed letters are now employed, the child tracing them with his hand held by the teacher, naming them, looking at them, repeating the name.

8. The next stage—word reading—is difficult from the impossibility of obtaining good carved combinations of sounds or raised word blocks, but by this time words printed under a picture, as in ordinary reading books, have generally become fairly intelligible, and the order look, speak, copy, write, is found useful.

It should be noted that the first block letter feeling is never given up, as it is obvious that this is the link which re-established connexion between the visual impression and the word Motor-Memory.

9. Without giving up the general curative practice, an attempt is now made to teach the child reading in the ordinary way. It is here that the school-teacher's help is most valuable; in the case of M.G. mentioned above it was extremely helpful and produced a rapid result.

The facility with which the normal 'word-blind' draw is very remarkable. They are generally far above the average of their age and in several instances they have followed the profession of art.

The suggestion left by these studies is that the path to re-establishment of normal conditions lies along a vigorous course of motor training associated with visual and auditive impression. In effect, a strong intensification of one stage in the normal child's approach to learning to read.

Glossary

ABNORMAL. Not normal; not conformable with nature or with the general rule.

ACQUIRED. Pertaining to some habit or disease which is not congenital.

> *a., character.* A change in one or more organs of the body which has occurred during the lifetime of the individual, and which is due to disease, or use, or misuse of the organ or organs so affected.

> *a., movements.* Those brought under the influence of the will only after conscious and attentive effort and practice, in distinction from re-acquired movements, those reinstated in their former proficiency after injury to the motor regions of the brain.

ACTIVE, PASSIVE, REACTIVE. Three descriptive types of mental attitude. Activity leads to expansion and expression, passivity leads to dormancy and stupidity, reactivity leads to neurosis or else to delinquency.

ACTUATION. The mental function that is exercised between the impulse of volition and its performance.

ADOLESCENCE. A period involving the change from childhood to adulthood occurring about the age of 12–21 (female) or 14–25 (male).

AFFERENT. Carrying towards the centre.

> *a., nerves.* Nerves conveying impulses towards the central nervous system.

AGNOSIA. Loss of the perceptive faculty which gives recognition of persons and things. The types correspond with the several senses and are distinguished as auditory, visual, gustatory, tactile, &c.

AGORAPHOBIA. A morbid fear of open places or spaces.

AGRAMMATISM. A phenomenon of Aphasia, consisting in the inability to form words grammatically or the suppression of certain words of a phrase.

AGRAPHIA. Inability to express ideas by writing.

> *a., absolute.* A variety in which no letters can be formed.
>
> *a., acoustic.* Loss of capacity to write from dictation.
>
> *a., amnemonica.* A form in which letters can be written, but without conveying any meaning.
>
> *a., atactica.* That form in which letters cannot be formed from lack of muscular co-ordination.
>
> *a., motor.* Inability to recall the movements of the hand necessary in writing.
>
> *a., musical.* Pathological loss of the ability to write musical notes.
>
> *a., optic.* Inability to copy writing, but ability to write from dictation.
>
> *a., verbal.* A variety in which a number of words without meaning can be written.

ALALIA. 1. Impairment of articulation from paralysis of the muscles of speech or from local laryngeal disease.

> 2. Aphasia due to a psychic disorder. Cf. *dyslalia, lalophobia, mogilalia, paralalia.*

ALEXIA. Word blindness. A form of Aphasia in which the patient is unable to recognize written or printed characters.

> *a., motor.* Inability to read aloud what is written or printed, although it is comprehended.
>
> *a., musical.* Loss of the ability to read music.
>
> *a., optic.* Inability to comprehend written or printed words.

AMENTIA. A condition in which the mind has failed to develop.

AMNESIA (forgetfulness). Loss of memory, especially of the ideas represented by words.

ANARTHRIA. Defective articulation.

APHASIA. Partial or complete loss of the power of expressing ideas by means of speech or writing. Aphasia may be either motor or sensory.

APHEMIA. Motor Aphasia; inability to articulate words of sentences from Centric and not from Peripheral disease.

APHONIA. Voicelessness due to loss of speech, due to some peripheral lesion, or to hysterical, or paralytic absence of the power of speech.

    a., Clericorum. Clergyman's sore throat.

    a., Paranoica. Stubborn silence in the mentally affected.

APHTHONGIA. Spasm of the muscles supplied by the hypoglossal nerve.

APRAXIA (abnormal clumsiness). Soul-blindness; mind-blindness; object blindness; an affection in which the memory for the uses of things is lost, as well as the understanding of the signs by which the things are expressed.

ASSIMILATION. The reduction of the movements of articulation. When two sounds come together the movements of articulation which are common to both are executed once only.

ASTEREOGNOSIS. Inability to recognize objects by the sense of touch, due to lesion in the central parietal lobule.

ATROPHY. Diminution in the size of a tissue, organ or part, the result of degeneration of the cells or a decrease in the size of the cells.

AUDITORY. Pertaining to the act or the organs of hearing.

AUTISTIC. To be self-absorbed, shut off from environment and preoccupied with internal thought.

AUTO-SUGGESTION. The technique by which an individual directs his unconscious depths according to the ideas and decisions he has consciously chosen. The arousal of an emotional tone in the self in agreement with intellectual conclusions, thus banishing conflict between thought and feeling. Also the acceptance by the individual without reflection of a proposition arising within the mind itself.

BABBLING (baby talk). The repetition of meaningless sounds.

BACKWARDNESS. The retardation of mental development through disease, sense-deprivation or other adverse causes.

BLINDNESS. Want of vision.

> *b., cortical.* Blindness due to lesion of the cortical centre of vision.
>
> *b., psychic.* Loss of conscious visual sensation from destruction of the cerebral visual centre; there is sight but not recognition. *See* ALEXIA.
>
> *b., object. See* APRAXIA.

BULIMIA. Excessive morbid hunger; it sometimes occurs in the mentally defective and the insane.

CENTRIC. Relating to a centre, especially to a nerve centre.

CEREBRAL. Relating to the cerebrum.

> *c., gyri.* The convolutions of the brain.
>
> *c., hemiplegia.* Hemiplegia due to cerebral apoplexy.
>
> *c., surprise.* The speedy but not long persistent stupor that often follows sudden mental shock or grave lesion or injury of the brain.
>
> *c., vesicles.* The embryonic vesicles from which the brain is developed.

CEREBRUM. The chief portion of the brain, occupying the whole upper part of the cranium, and consisting of the right and left hemispheres.

CHOREA (St. Vitus' dance). A functional nervous disorder, usually occurring in youth, characterized by irregular and involuntary action of the muscles of the extremities, face, &c., with general muscular weakness. Rheumatism often co-exists. Chorea may be caused by a number of conditions, among which are fright and reflex irritation. It affects girls about three times as frequently as boys.

    c., *laryngeal*. (i) A condition attended with clonic spasm of the laryngeal muscles and marked by inability to sustain co-ordinate action.

             (ii) A condition marked by spasmodic motions of some of the muscles of expiration, causing a cry.

    c., *imitative*. Choreic movements developed in children from association with choreic subjects.

CLAUSTROPHOBIA. Morbid fear of confined spaces.

CLINICAL. (i) Relating to bedside treatment or to a clinic.

        (ii) Pertaining to the symptoms and course of a disease as observed by the physician, in opposition to the anatomical changes found by the pathologist.

CLUTTERING. Hurried jumbled speech.

CONGENITAL. Existing at birth.

CO-ORDINATION. The harmonious activity and proper sequence of operation of those parts that co-operate in the performance of any function.

CORTEX. The outer surface of the brain which contains the nerve cells and most of their inter-connexions. It is the cortex which is referred to as the 'grey matter' of the brain.

CRETINISM. A congenital disease, characterized by the absence of the thyroid gland, diminutiveness of size, thickness of neck, shortness of arms and legs, prominence of abdomen, large size of face, thickness of lips, large and protruding tongue and imbecility or idiocy. It occurs endemically in the goitrous districts of Switzerland, and sporadically in other parts of Europe and in America. Lack of the secretion of the thyroid gland seems to be the cause.

DEAF. Entire lack of the sense of hearing; also impaired hearing.

d., fields. Two small triangular planes, which converge towards the external auditory meatus, and in which the vibrating tuning-fork is not heard.

d., mutism. Both deaf and dumb; the deafness may be congenital or acquired, and prevent the person from learning to speak.

d., points. Some points near the ear where a vibrating tuning-fork cannot be heard.

DEAFNESS. Due to disease of the external auditory canal, the middle ear, the internal ear, the auditory nerve, or the brain.

d., bass. Difficulty in hearing low tones.

d., cerebral. That due to a brain lesion.

d., cortical. That due to disease of the cortical hearing centres.

d., mind, d., psychic. Inability to recognize the sounds heard, due to the destruction of the central area of the auditory centre.

d., speech. A variety of psychic deafness resembling word deafness, except that the faculty of repeating and writing after dictation is not lost.

d., tone (tone-deafness). Sensory amusia.

d., word. See *psychic deafness.*

DEMENTIA. A form of insanity characterized by a deteriorization or loss of the intellectual faculties, the reasoning power, the memory, and the will.

d., paralytic. General paralysis of the insane.

d., paranoides. A form of *d. praecox*, characterized by paranoiac delusions.

d., praecox. A dementia more or less complete which appears at the age of puberty in those previously intellectually bright. There is an upset physiological equilibrium with low metabolic rate, low blood pressure, low pulse rate and waste fluid output.

d., primary. That occurring independently of other forms of insanity.

d., *secondary*. That following another form of insanity.

d., *senile*. That due to degenerations of old age.

d., *terminal*. That coming on towards the end of other forms of insanity or certain nervous diseases.

DEVELOPMENTAL. Incidental to growth. This term is used to describe that condition where the disorder, although due to hereditary and congenital causes, does not manifest itself until the stage has been reached where certain characteristics should normally appear.

DYSENEIA. Disorders of articulation due to deafness.
(American Speech Correction Association)

DYSLALIA. An acute form of lisping and lalling accompanied by complete or partial disco-ordination of the muscles governing speech.

DYSPHASIA. Difficulty in speech depending on central lesion.

DYSPHEMIA. Stammering.

DYPHONIA. Partial loss of voice.

DYSPHORIA. Impatience and restlessness; mental anxiety; fidgets.

DYSPHRASIA. Imperfect speech due to impairment of mental power.

DYSPHRENIA. Any mental disorder.

ECHOLALIA. A meaningless repetition of words and phrases.

EFFERENT. Carrying away.

e., *nerves*. Nerves conveying impulses away from the central nervous system.

EMBRYO. The germ of an organism before it has developed its distinctive form.

ENCEPHALITIS. Inflammation of the brain.

e., *lethargia*. An epidemic form of encephalitis frequently occurring with influenza and characterized by drowsiness, apathy, muscular weakness and paralysis of the third cranium nerve. It is sometimes diagnosed at the outset as influenza.

e., periaxialia diffusa. A disease mostly of children. It manifests itself by marked loss of hearing, speech and sight; due to cerebral inflammation.

ENDOCRINE GLANDS. Ductless glands, or the glands of internal secretion.

ENURESIS (bed-wetting). Incontinence of urine.

ERYTHROMANIA. Compulsive blushing.

EUPHORIA. A feeling of well-being.

EXHIBITIONISM. Gratification through exposing the body or showing off the mind.

EXTROVERT. One whose mind is predominately extroverted.

EXTROVERSION. The turning of one's interests outward towards the world of reality.

FACULTY. A special action of the mind through the instrumentality of an organ or organs.

FAUCES (the upper part of the throat). The space surrounded by the palate, tonsils and uvula.

FEEBLE-MINDEDNESS (high-grade Amentia).

> Persons in whose case there exists from birth or from an early age mental defectiveness not amounting to imbecility, yet so pronounced that they require care, supervision, and control for their own protection or for the protection of others, or in the case of children, that they, by reason of such defectiveness, appear to be permanently incapable of receiving proper benefit from the instruction in ordinary schools.—(Mental Deficiency Act, 1913.)

FIBRIL. A name applied to minute nerve filaments.

FIBRILLARY CONTRACTIONS. Spontaneous contractions successively taking place in different bundles of muscular fibres.

FRICATIVE. Made by friction of breath in narrow opening. When the current of air passing through the mouth is partially stopped and does not completely cut off the sound.

FUNCTIONAL. Pertaining to the special action of an organ.

FUNCTIONAL DISORDERS OF SPEECH. Those due to imperfect perception of speech or imperfect control of the process of utterance, in spite of normal organs of speech.

GESTATION. Pregnancy.
GYRUS. A convolution of the brain.

HEMIATROPHY. Atrophy confined to one side of the body.
HEMIPLEGIA. Paralysis of one side of the body.
HYPER. Excessive, e.g. hyper-rhinolalia, excessive nasality.
HYPERTROPHY. An increase in the size of a tissue or organ, independent of the general growth of the body.
HYPO. Lack of, e.g. hypo-rhinolalia, inadequate nasality.

IDIOGLOSSIA. Extremely defective utterance, but one in which the same sound is used to express the same idea, even though the sound used belongs to no known language.
IDIOT. A person congenitally almost destitute of intelligence.
IMBECILES (medium-grade Amentia).

Persons in whose case there exists from birth or from an early age mental defectiveness not amounting to idiocy, yet so pronounced that they are incapable of managing themselves or their affairs, or, in the case of children, of being taught to do so.—(Mental Deficiency Act, 1913.)

INFERIORITY COMPLEX. An inferiority in some particular respect, for which the person tries unconsciously to compensate by exaggerated efforts to prove superiority in some other respect.
INHIBITION. The act of checking or restraining. The checking of one nervous impulse by another.
INNERVATION. A discharge of nervous force.
INSTINCT. A natural impulse, which, though unassociated with reason, prompts a useful act.
INTELLIGENCE QUOTIENT (I.Q.). The ratio between an individual's mental age and his chronological age multiplied by 100. Normal mentality would therefore be 100.
INTERDENTAL. Between the teeth.

INTROVERT. One whose mind is predominantly self-centred; one whose thought is centripetal or egocentric.

INVERSION (in the psychological sense). The principle by which the defence mechanism of neurosis makes a person masquerade as his opposite; as the superiority pose of some forms of inferiority feeling.

KINOESTHESIS. Sensations from the muscles, tendons and joints by which muscular motion, weight, position, &c., are perceived. It is from these sensations that new patterns of movement are largely established.

KYPHO-LORDOSIS. *See* LORDOSIS.

LABIAL (as applied to speech). Sounds in which movements or position of the lips play a part, such as p, b, m.

LALIA. Speech.

LALLING. Baby talk.

LALONEUROSIS. An impairment of speech arising from spasmodic action of the muscles.

LALOPATHY. Any disorder of speech.

LALOPHOBIA. Stutter-spasm, leading to or complicated with a dislike of speaking.

LISPING. A defeat of speech in which sibilant letters are sounded like linguals, especially a and th.

    a., *neurotic lisping*, a form of lisping allied to a nervous inhibition which shows itself in an uncontrolled spasm on the sound affected.

    b., *lateral lisp*. A severe form of nervous lisping accompanied by severe facial spasm. The effect appears like paralysis.

    c., *organic lisp*. Lisping due to some injury, malformation, disease or degeneration of the organs of speech.

    d., *sigmatism*. Defective utterance of the 's' sound.

LOGAGNOSIA. Aphasia.

LOGAGRAPHIA. Same as agraphia.

LOGAMNESIA. Forgetfulness.

II

LOGAPHASIA. Aphasia for lack of articulation.

LOGO. A prefix meaning relating to word or speech.

LOGOPATHY. A disease affecting the speech.

LOGORRHEA. Excessive loquacity.

LORDOSIS. A forward curvature of the spine.

MACROCEPHALY. Abnormal largeness of the head.

MASOCHISM. Gratification, sometimes of a sexual nature, derived from being cruelly treated.

MASTURBATION. Sexual self-abuse.

MEGALOMANIA. Delusion of greatness.

MENTAL DEFICIENCY. Imperfect development of the mental faculties due to incomplete development of the nerve cells of the brain.

METABOLISM. The transformation of foodstuffs into living matter and the breaking down of living matter into simpler products within a cell or organism.

MICROCEPHALY. Abnormal smallness of the head.

MONGOLIAN IDIOCY. A type of idiocy having some similarities to myxoedema and cretinism; the face is broad, nose flat or stubby, eyes obliquely set, mouth open, skin fat and soft, muscles flaccid.

MORBID. Diseased, pathological.

MORON. A child with permanently arrested mental development; but of higher grade than an imbecile.

MOTIVES. Basic impulses.

MUTISM. Failure, or inability to talk.

MYOTONIA. 1. Tonic muscular spasm.
2. The stretching of a muscle.

NASALITY. A peculiar muffled timbre of the voice, especially marked in cases of perforated palate. (*See* RHINO-PHONIA.)

NEGATIVISM. An attitude of opposition towards the suggestion or commands of others.

NEURASTHENIA. A group of symptoms resulting from debility or exhaustion of the nerve centres.

NEUROBLAST. A cell derived from the primitive ectoderm, and giving rise to nerve fibres and nerve cell.

NEUROLOGY. A speciality in medicine dealing with diseases of the nervous system, especially in their physical aspects.

NEURONE. One of the countless number of units of which the nervous system is composed. Each neuron consists of a cell and a series of processes. In every physiological act involving the nervous system at least two, usually more, neurons participate. The neuron at which the impulse starts is termed archineuron; the one at the termination teleneuron.

NEUROSIS. Any morbid nervous state. A functional disease of the neurons system, a disturbance of the nerve centres or peripheral nerves not due to any demonstrable structural change.

NEUROTIC LISP. (*See* LISPING.)

OBSESSION. A dominant delusion. A compulsive idea which is inaccessible to reason.

OBTURATOR. That which closes an opening.

OCCLUSIVE. Closing or shutting up, occlusive consonant. A complete breath stop.

ONOMATOMANIA. Functional derangement of speech, of which five varieties are described:

    (*a*) A powerful effort to recall a word.

    (*b*) An irresistible impulse continually to repeat a word by which the patient seems perplexed.

    (*c*) The patient attaches some peculiar meaning to a commonplace word.

    (*d*) The patient repeats certain words as a safeguard.

    (*e*) The patient is impelled to spit out some word, like a disgusting morsel.

ORAL. Pertaining to the mouth, the organs of speech— spoken word.

ORBICULAR—circular. As the orbicular muscle of the eye or mouth.

11*

ORGANIC. Pertaining to any part of the body having a definite function to perform.

ORTHODONTICS. 'That branch of dentistry which deals with the principles and practices involved in the prevention and correction of malocclusion of the teeth, and such other malformations and abnormalities as may be associated therewith.'

PALATAL DEFECTS. All disorders of speech pertaining to the palate.

PARALYSIS. A loss of motion or of sensation in a part.

PARANOIA. Mental aberration, especially a chronic disease characterized by systematized delusions.

PARAPHASIA. A form of Aphasia in which there is inability to connect ideas with the proper words to express ideas.

PARAPHEMIA. Paraphasia in which the same words are often used wrongly.

PARAPHONIA. Any abnormal condition of the voice.

    p., *claugens*. Shrillness of the voice.

    p., *puberum*. The harsh, deep, irregular voice noticed in boys at puberty.

PARAPHRASIA. A form of Aphasia characterized by incoherence of speech.

PARAPHRENIA. Delirium. A mental disease.

PARESIS. A slight paralysis; incomplete loss of muscular power.

PATHOLOGICAL. Pertaining to disease.

PERCEPTION. The process of acquiring knowledge through the senses.

PETIT MAL. A slight epileptic attack.

PHANTASY. Dream-living. The act of withdrawal from the world and building in place of actuality another world within the depths of the mind.

PHILOLOGY. Science of the structure and development of language.

PHOBIA. An abnormal fear.

PHONAESTHENIA. Weak whispered tone. Physical sensibility. Sense awareness through the senses.

PHONATION. The production of vocal sound or articulate speech. (*See* HYPO and HYPER.)

PHONOPATHY. Any disorder or disease of the voice.

PHONOPHOBIA. 1. A fear of speaking in paraesthesia of the larynx, because of the painful sensation produced during phonation.

2. Morbid dread of any sound or noise.

PLANTIGRADE. Bringing the entire length of the sole of the foot to the ground in walking, as is seen in the bear.

PROGNOSIS. An opinion or judgement in advance concerning the duration, course, and termination of a disease.

PROPHYLAXIS. Prevention of disease; measures preventing the development or spread of disease.

PSYCHOGENESIS. The development of mental characteristics.

PSYCHOGENETIC. Of psychic or mental origin.

PSYCHOGENIC. (Disorders of speech.) Those of psychic and mental origin. Disorders due to nervous disturbances.

PSYCHONEUROSIS. Mental disease independent of organic lesion.

PSYCHOPATHY. Any disease of the mind.

PSYCHOSIS. A disease of the mind, especially one without demonstrable organic lesions. Any morbid mental state.

PUBERTY. The age of sexual maturity.

PYREXIA. Fever. Elevation of temperature above the normal.

PYROMANIA. A monomania for incendiarism (the impulse to set fire to things).

RELAXATION. A diminution of tension in a part; a diminution in functional activity.

RHINOLALIA. A nasal tone in the voice due to undue closure (rhinolalia clausa) or to undue patulousness (rhinolalia aperta) of the posterior nares.

RHINOPHONIA. A nasal tone in speaking.

  Hyper-rhiniphonia. Excessive nasality.

  Hypo-rhinophonia. Inadequate nasality.

SADISM. Pleasure derived from inflicting cruelty on others.

SCANNING. A peculiar slow and measured form of speech, occurring in various nervous affections.

SCHIZOPHRENIA. Dementia praecox, or more especially the splitting up of personality characteristic of praecox cases.

SEPTUM. A partition; a division wall. Nasal septum, the septum between the two nasal cavities.

SIBILANT. Consonants having a hissing sound—as s, z, sh and c.

SIGMATISM. Difficulty with the 's' sound.

SINUSITIS. Inflammation of a sinus.

SPASM. A sudden muscular contraction.

    s., clonic. A spasm broken by relaxation of the muscles.

    s., tonic. A spasm that persists without relaxation for some time.

SPEECH MECHANISM. The whole of the machinery concerned in speech.

STAMMERING. A nervous disturbance affecting speech.

STIGMATA (of degeneracy). Physical signs most commonly seen in the mentally abnormal or defective.

SUPERIORITY COMPLEX. Arrogant pride.

STREPHIOSYMBOLIA (word blindness).

Difficulty in learning to read.

Tendency to reverse the direction of reading.

SYNDROME. The aggregate symptoms of a disease; a complex of symptoms.

TETANY. A disease characterized by intermittent lilateral, painful, tonic spasms of the muscles, specially of the upper extremities.

THERAPEUTICS. The branch of medicine dealing with the treatment and curing of disease.

TIC. A muscular spasm or twitching, often of the facial muscles.

TOXIC. Poisonous.

TRAUMA. A severe wound or injury, or in the psychic realm, an experience of painful emotional character.

TURBINATED—Top-shaped; scroll-shaped.

> *t., bone.* One of the three (superior, middle, and inferior) bony projections upon the outer wall of each nasal fossa. They are covered by an erectile vascular mucous membrane.

UVULA. The conical appendix hanging from the free edge of the soft palate and formed by muscles, mucous membrane and connective tissue.

UVULITIS. Inflammation of the uvula, causing loss of voice and acute discomfort.

VELUM PALATI. The soft palate. Velum pendulum palate, the soft palate, especially the uvula.

VISUAL. Of, or concerned with, or used in seeing.

VOLITION. The faculty of will by which the powers are directed towards the attainment of a chosen end.

Bibliography

Adler, Alfred. *Understanding Human Nature.*
Aikin, W. A. *The Voice.*
Association of Education Committee Report, 1933.
Asquith, Lady Cynthia. *The King's Daughters.*

Boome, E. J., and Richardson, M. A. *The Nature and Treatment of Stammering.*
        Relaxation in Everyday Life.
Boome, E. J. *Some Aspects of Stammering.* (Mental Welfare, Oct., 1934.)
        The Difficult Child. (The Teacher of the Deaf, June, 1934.)
        Speech Defects in Young Children. (Public Health, 1937.)
        Cause and Modern Treatment of Speech Disorders. (Journal of the Royal Sanitary Institute, 1937.)
British Museum Publications, Set B. 49. *Masks from Ceylon.*
Bühler, C. *The Mental Development of the Child.*
Burt, Cyril. *The Young Delinquent.*
        The Backward Child.
Butler, W. Bowden. *The Book of Margery Kempe.*

Cameron, H. C. *The Nervous Child.*
Carpenter, C. D. Hale. *A Naturalist on Lake Victoria.*
Compton, J. *Spoken English.*

Dixon, Macneile. *The Human Situation.*

Data of Child Development. (Publication No. 91 Children's Bureau U.S. Department of Labour.)
Duncan, J. *Mental Deficiency*.

Ewing, A. W. G. *Aphasia in Childhood*.

Fogerty, Elsie. *First Notes on Speech Training*.
        Speech Craft.
        Rhythm.
        Notes on Some Cases of Word Blindness. (The Journal of Speech Disorders.)
Fröschels, E. *Das Stottern*.
        Twentieth Century Speech and Voice Correction.

Goldstein. *The After Effects of Brain Injuries in War*.
Gordon Smith, A. *Short History of Medieval England*.
Gordon, Sir George. *Shakespeare's English*. (S.P.E. Tract XXIX.)

Haeckel, Ernst. *The Riddle of the Universe*.
Halls, Emily Clegg. *Indiana Survey for Children Handicapped in Speech*. (The Indiana Teacher, April, 1936.)
Hart, B. *Psychology of Insanity*.
Head, H. *Aphasia*.
Herbert, A. P. *What a Word!*
Hocart, A. M. *The Progress of Man*.

Jacobson. *Progressive Relaxation*.
Johnson, Wendell. *Because I Stutter*.

Kingdon-Ward, W. *Stammering*.

Lewis, M. M. *Infant Speech*.

McAllister, A. H. *Clinical Studies in Speech Therapy*.
Mandell, A. E. *Psychology for Every Man (and Woman)*.
Morley, Muriel E. *Cleft Palate and Speech*.

Negus, V. E. *The Mechanism of the Larynx*.

Orton, S. T. *Reading, Writing and Speech Problems in Children*.

Paget, Sir Richard. *Human Speech*.

Ripman, W. *Sounds of Spoken English*.
Ripon, T. S., and Fletcher, Peter. *Reassurance and Relaxation*.
Ripper, Harold. *Vital Speech*.

Schonell, F. J. *The Relationship between Defective Speech and Disability in Spelling*. (Journal of Educational Psychology, June, 1934.)
Seth, George, and Guthrie, Douglas. *Speech in Childhood*.
Sheridan, Mary D., M.D., L.R.A.M. *The Child's Hearing for Speech*.
Shrubsall, F. C., and Williams, A. C. *Mental Deficiency Practice*.
Sollas, W. T. *Ancient Hunters*.
Stein, Leopold. *Speech and Voice*.
                 Infancy of Speech.
Stern, W. *Psychology of Early Childhood*. Trans. by A. Barwell.

Tredgold, A. F. *Mental Deficiency*.

van Thal, Joan H. *Cleft Palate Speech*.
                 The Relationship between Faults of Dentition and Defects of Speech. (The Proceedings of the Second International Congress of Phonetic Sciences.)

Ward, I. C. *Defects of Speech*.
Wedberg, Conrad F. *The Stutterer Speaks*.
West, R., Kennedy, Lou, and Carr, Anna. *Rehabilitation of Speech*.

Index

Note : G = Glossary

Printed in Great Britain by Butler & Tanner Ltd., Frome and London